Covid-19 & Post Covid-19 Alleviate the Fear

Dr. Rodica Malos, DNP

TRILOGY CHRISTIAN PUBLISHERS

TUSTIN, CA

Trilogy Christian Publishers
A Wholly Owned Subsidiary of Trinity Broadcasting Network
2442 Michelle Drive
Tustin, CA 92780

For information, address Trilogy Christian Publishing

Rights Department, 2442 Michelle Drive, Tustin, Ca 92780.

Trilogy Christian Publishing/ TBN and colophon are trademarks of Trinity Broadcasting Network.

For information about special discounts for bulk purchases, please contact Trilogy Christian Publishing.

Manufactured in the United States of America

Trilogy Disclaimer: The views and content expressed in this book are those of the author and may not necessarily reflect the views and doctrine of Trilogy Christian Publishing or the Trinity Broadcasting Network.

10 9 8 7 6 5 4 3 2 1

Library of Congress Cataloging-in-Publication Data is available.
ISBN 978-1-63769-194-6
ISBN 978-1-63769-195-3 (ebook)

Contents

Disclaimer

This book contains the opinions and ideas of its author and does not reflect the point of view of the organization or the clinic mentioned in this book. It is solely for informational and educational purposes and should not be regarded as a substitute for professional medical treatment. You as a reader should NOT USE any medication mentioned in this book without medical advice. The nature of your body's health condition is complex and unique. Therefore, you should consult a health professional before you begin any new lifestyle change, exercise, nutrition, fasting, or supplementation program, or if you have questions about your health. Neither the author nor the publisher shall be liable or responsible for any loss or damage allegedly arising from any information or suggestion in this book. People and names in this book are composites created by the author from her experiences as a primary care practitioner. Names and details of their stories have been changed, and any similarity between the names and stories of individuals

Endorsements

Ever since the pandemic began there have been many articles and even books written. Unfortunately, many of them created more confusion than clarity for the avid reader. This was due partly to their lack of appeal to all of the implications created by the COVID-19 pandemic. This book has the advantage of addressing all of the aspects related to the impact of COVID-19 on people. Dr. Malos writes from the perspective of a scholar, with the passion of a physician and the spiritual insight of a Christian.

Although she is not writing from her office in the academic ivory tower of a scholar, her book is very well researched, with plenty of quotations from reputable scholars in the medical field. Rather, the book seems to have been written between the walls of her clinic while in touch with the reality of the suffering provoked by the pandemic. Therefore, she is not afraid to go against mainstream medical recommendations and recommend the right treatment for her patients and readers.

Dr. Malos' more than thirty years' experience in the medical field has helped her to truly understand the struggles of those infected with the virus and the heavy impact on their well-being. Nevertheless, the great advantage of this book is its spiritual perspective. As a university professor and pastor, I can understand how important it is to address the spiritual impact of the pandemic on people. By approaching the pandemic from a holistic perspective—physical, emotional and spiritual—the author is giving readers hope not only for a better life on this earth, but a new perspective on eternal life! I highly recommend this book to anyone who wants to learn how to treat and deal with COVID-19!

Crinisor Stefan, PhD

Pastor - Agape Christian Church, Yorba Linda, CA

Adjunct Faculty, Vanguard University, Costa Mesa, CA

"He that dwelleth in the secret place of the most High shall abide under the shadow of the Almighty... Surely he shall deliver thee... from the noisome pestilence... Thou shalt not be afraid for the terror by night... nor for the pestilence that walketh in darkness; nor for destruction that wasteth at noonday" (Psalm 91:1-6 KJV).

The writer's faith in God as the Protector carries her through the challenges of the COVID-19 pandemic by turning her to help and assist many sick people. She identifies and confronts her fear of the unprecedented and unpredictable virus spread. Supplied by amazing, emotional, biblical support and vast knowledge derived from the tireless research she has conducted, the author becomes a gentle healing tool in the loving hands of Jehovah Rapha. The outcome consists of saved lives and souls for the eternal kingdom.

The book encouraged me personally to supersede the fear, just like Dr. Rodica Malos has done in the writing of this book, and to consecrate myself to Almighty God. By cosigning our lives and wisdom to His almighty protection, we will survive.

Dr. Mihaela Beloiu, Senior MD
NWKP Family Practice
Portland, Oregon

COVID-19 hit hard in the twenty-first century and found the world so unprepared! Rodica stood against the wave with courage and took the risk of being exposed to COVID-19, only to walk in Jesus' footsteps. Not tormented by the coronavirus, she went forward, equipped with the Word of God, studying and discerning medical literature, devoted to suffering people while keeping her eyes on the Great Physician. And as such, she has had a great impact on the community!

This is not a theoretical textbook! Instead, Rodica, using her ability to discern the lesser from the greater, works hard and gathers insights, supported by her medical experiences and information from several medical experts. She has real stories to tell, and testimonies which bloom with hope and encouragement.

There is practical wisdom embroidered in her pages. She is pointing constantly at the Great Physician, Jesus, who offers not changing theories but the absolute truth. The Great Healer in town can examine you thoroughly and make you whole, in the midst of the pandemic storm!

Just don't miss the appointment with Him! Stay equipped!

Dr. Crisan Crisan-Dume, MD
Diplomate of American Board of Family Medicine,
Urgent Care
Vancouver, WA

Doctor Rodica Malos is a well-known and trusted member of our community. Through this book, she gives the reader a perspective not shared by many of us.

Like many other doctors, she could have taken a much easier way through the pandemic by following the passive approach: to isolate herself and her potential patients, embracing the "sicken-in-place" paradigm. However, as a believer in God and in His Word, Doctor Malos knew that the implications of COVID-19 infections went far beyond fever, sneezing, dry cough, etc. She knew that more than ever, any person who tested positive or was exposed to the virus needed to find hope and to escape the poisonous effects of fear, in addition to physical healing.

Motivated by compassion and moved by the increased number of cries for help, Doctor Rodica Malos, with care and passion, developed the best available early intervention methods for at-home care, preventing the hospitalization of hundreds of people in the Romanian community as well as many underserved members of racial and ethnic minority groups in our region.

This book is a must read for everyone who seeks to understand the complex set of implications of a pandemic, or any other kind of life-threatening event which may occur in the future. As a pastor, I believe the most outstanding merit of this book is the fact that Doctor Rodica Malos shares her perspective on the essential role of faith and the church, to counter the feeling of helplessness when confronted with life-and-death situations. The reader gets the opportunity to examine their own relationship with God and with His Son, Jesus, whom the author presents as the true source of healing and peace.

I am ecstatic to recommend to you the latest book from Doctor Rodica Malos, to discover for yourself a practical path to spiritual, emotional, and physical health.

Rev. Vasile Cinpean,
Lead Pastor—Philadelphia Romanian Church,
Portland, Oregon
President of the Romanian Alliance Assemblies of
God, USA

Dr. Rodica Malos has written an eye-opening, personal account of a primary care provider's experience of struggles, questions, frustrations, criticisms, and ultimately deliverance with discernment, wisdom, and joy, while trying to provide the best care for her patients during a confusing pandemic with flip-flopping national and state emergency measures varying by state. This comprehensive, scholarly, and Scripture-filled book, written in the midst of the global COVID-19 pandemic by a well-trained frontline primary care provider, shares many helpful answers for the reader and provides evidence-based therapies not widely disseminated; more importantly, the book points to a great and living hope with redemptive peace for those under great stress and fear, including those who mourn the loss of loved ones. I was inspired by her personal experience of seeking discernment and wisdom on how to best care for her despairing, sickened patients from the only gracious, loving, omniscient, omnipotent Healer and Giver of Life.

Dr. Rodica shares the discoveries of her compassionate, diligent search for meaning and for the answers to the many questions from her own desperate patients, who found few answers and little comfort from the overwhelmed health care system that seemed to prescribe certain treatments in favor of "sickening in place" until requiring hospitalization. She addresses her patients' depression and anxiety, aggravated by mandated lockdown orders causing isolation, prohibition of communities of faith from in-person gathering and mutual support (even when abiding by social distancing and mask orders), and the resultant widespread economic hardship.

Her search for valid information to help her patients was further hindered by politically motivated misinformation and censorship of data. Fear and criticism from other providers unfamiliar with the available data— not only from the USA, but internationally—was another potential discourager. Yet because of Dr Malos' tenacious compassion, faithful perseverance, and trust in the One who is Sovereign even over a coronavirus, she has been given the mantle to present the rewarding results of her well-documented observational study of treating her early symptomatic COVID-19 infected patients. This account of a dedicated doctor carefully pursuing the available evidence, guided by her faith in her omniscient Heavenly Father, is to the praise of His glory indeed!

"Incline my heart to Your testimonies, and not to covetousness. Turn away my eyes from looking at worthless things, and revive me in Your way. Establish Your word to Your servant, who is devoted to fearing You" (Psalm 119:36-38 NKJV).

Dr. Robert Saysoon, MD
Diplomate of American Board of Internal Medicine
Portland, Oregon

I thank God for this book of wisdom, where faith takes fear captive. Dr. Malos dissects divine science with regard to our response to the global coronavirus pandemic. Her plan to emphasize prevention and to promote wellness utilizes existing best practices and existing standards of care.

Deviating from these only produces failure and chaos. Let us take heart that there are practitioners who choose life and inject this pandemic with solid spiritual insight, knowledge, wisdom, and compassion. Their gift of discernment and a sound mind truly advances the health of the entire planet.

Kay E. Metsger, RN, BSN
Former Cardiac Nurse Manager
Cardiac Operating Room
Providence St. Vincent Hospital and Medical
Center
Portland, Oregon

Dr. Malos offers exceptional insight into outpatient treatment protocols for COVID-19 and highlights the lifesaving and disease mitigating properties of these regimens. The failure to implement such measures will be deemed one of the greatest failures of medicine in the 21st century. I applaud Dr. Malos' courage and efforts to intervene on behalf of her patients. Well done!

Naomi R. Florea, Pharm.D.
Co-Founder, Infectious Disease Specialist
Choice Care Concierge Medicine
Costa Mesa, California

"In this book, Dr. Maloş shares her experiences as a frontline medical practitioner. It is very practical and full of much helpful information. She gives medical as well as spiritual solutions for dealing with the COVID-19 pandemic. This includes medications and treatment protocols as well as strategies for dealing with anxiety, fear, and depression. It provides a very balanced and holistic approach. I recommend this book to everyone who wants to learn how to navigate this worldwide pandemic successfully."

Oliver Ghitea, MD
Anesthesiologist
Portland, Oregon

Acknowledgements

This book received support from the Creator of the universe, who gave the world supernatural prescriptions in His living Word to overcome fear and to manage high levels of stress, anxiety, and depression during pandemic time and every day in life. I thank Jesus Christ, the Lord and Savior of my life and the entire world, the Lamb of God, who delivers those who believe in Him from the stress of sin and from all their fears in any situation including pandemic time. Only He restores the joy of salvation, and gives hope, and peace that passes all understanding and guards their minds, spirits, and bodies during this pandemic period.

I acknowledge the Holy Spirit, the great Comforter, who literally guided every step in treating patients with symptoms from Covid-19 and in writing this book. He is the Power of God working on Earth, giving to those who ask Him inspiration, wisdom, knowledge, revelation, and discernment to cope with high levels of stress, fear, anxiety, and depression. Also, I give millions of

thanks to my beloved husband, Stelica, for his sacrifices, support, encouragement, and love during the pandemic, while I was involved extra hours in helping the
most vulnerable people suffering from symptoms from
Covid-19 at every level. Millions of thanks to my entire
family including the in-laws who worked in health care
on front line providing care relentlessly and tirelessly
to patients suffering from many kinds of diseases during the pandemic making great sacrifice. I give many
thanks to all friends, colleagues, and all my patients
who were in my sphere of influence and who provided
support and inspiration throughout the entire time
during pandemic.

Many thanks to all the writers, doctors, experts and
scientists cited in this book and all those standing for
the truth and the churches ("spiritual clinics") that continued to pray fervently for those in great need for healing. You sacrifice your time to make the information
available, to inspire me and the entire community. We
benefit from the scientific evidence and your spiritual
insights. You change our thinking and motivate us to
have a better lifestyle, to live a quality life here on earth
and for eternity. Special thanks to the entire team of
editors and Trilogy publisher at TBN for helping me
finish and publish this book. Special thanks to you for
reading the information in this book with the hope that
will enrich your knowledge and will give a new per-

spective for life on this planet and in eternity. It will strengthen your spirit, renew your mind and thoughts, improve your physical and spiritual health, and prevent physical and spiritual diseases.

PART I

CHAPTER 1

Overwhelming News

The Spirit of Fear and Sadness

"For God gave us a spirit not of fear but of power and love and self-control" (2 Timothy 1:7 ESV).

Over the past twelve months (at the time I am writing this book) we have heard on the local, national, and international news; on TV, internet, social media, newspaper, and radio; in stores, at work, and in conversations with professionals, friends, relatives, and family; that the most-used word is "COVID-19," and it is overwhelming and extremely stressful for everybody, instilling fear in people's minds and spirits. Fear is the greatest enemy of our health, physically and spiritually. Emotions of fear will stir up negative thoughts that will lead to anxiety and sadness, causing a shift in neurotransmitters and neurochemicals released in our body as serotonin, dopamine, melatonin, and other neurochemical levels decrease and further cause depression. That further will cause lack of sleep, leading to sleep deprivation, which weakens the immune system. I have learned my entire life that faith is the antidote to fear.

Dr. David Levy, MD, the best neurosurgeon in the world, talks in his video *Fear in Crisis - Part 1 (Help for Coronavirus COVID-19) Overcoming Anxiety* about how fear does affect people's brains, the immune system, and the entire body during a pandemic time. He explains how fear triggers thoughts and emotions that send signals to the brain that a danger is coming and send messages to the pituitary gland, which starts the process of secreting adrenocorticotropic hormones, stimulating the adrenal gland to release cortisol and epinephrine. The heart rate increases when stress from fear increases. The most dangerous is the cortisol that suppresses the immune system. The immune system helps the body to fight against bacteria, microorganisms, and viruses. Thoughts of fear and the emotions created by fear increase the chances of getting the virus by lowering the immune system that fights COVID-19.[1]

The Thoughts of Fear Are Poison

The thoughts of fear are poison for the mind and the body. Thoughts of fear occupy our mind and take up "real estate" in our brain with billions of neurons, and when we continue to repeat those thoughts of fear in our mind throughout the day, fear will control our mind. This causes the immune system to weaken and not be able to fight the virus COVID-19, and causes more damage to our body, soul, and spirit. Spiritually, we know who wants to destroy our life with thoughts of fear from uncertainty. In John 10:10 we read, "The thief does not come except to steal, and to kill, and to destroy. I have come that they may have life, and that they may have it more abundantly" (John 10:10 NKJV). I have come to the understanding that the battle is real in our mind through thoughts of fear and despair.

Fear and panic, stirred by the "invisible enemy" COVID-19, lead to increased levels of stress that cause an increase in cortisol (the stress hormone) and other neurotransmitters, affecting our mind and the ability to think and to make decisions. All body systems are affected by an unhealthy amount of neurochemicals released in the body during this stressful time. All systems connected to our brain are affected by increased levels of stress from fear, causing depression with all its consequences.

Mary Van Beusekom stated that "COVID-19 has tripled the rate of depression in US adults in all demographic groups—especially in those with financial worries—and the rise is much higher than after previous major traumatic events, according to a study published yesterday in *JAMA Network Open*."[2]

All of the people I talked to during this pandemic and patients with COVID-19 expressed fear, worry, anxiety, and reported thoughts of depression when we interacted on a regular basis during their sickness and disease.

COVID-19's Unpredictability

What I am writing in this book is what I have learned since January 22, 2020, when the first case of COVID-19 (a novel coronavirus named SARS-CoV-2 that originated in Wuhan, China in December 2019) was reported in the USA—and in those long months afterward—not only from the news, social media, the internet, online, in books, articles, papers, and the CDC, etc., but also from the struggles experienced by the patients with COVID-19 in our community.

For the most part, I learned from my own experience by taking care of patients with COVID-19 in an outpatient setting as a general practitioner in a small clinic in our area, with a mission to "provide excellent physical, mental, and spiritual care to the underserved with the love of Christ," where currently I volunteer my time to provide care to minority and needy people with many sicknesses and diseases. In more than two decades volunteering in a primary care setting, providing care to the most vulnerable population with acute and chronic health conditions, I never imagined that I would be one of the thousands of providers providing early care to outpatients suffering from the disease caused by CO-VID-19 during a pandemic time.

Always, my heart has been moved with compassion for those who suffer physically and psychologically from different illnesses—and now from the unpredictable COVID-19 and post COVID-19 virus symptoms.

When the discussion about the virus started in the USA in the beginning of the year 2020, like many medical providers, I was convinced that this was "another virus" that we would be able to control with our advanced knowledge in science, medicine, and advanced technology in pharmacology. I did not have doubts at that time that the COVID-19 virus would be controlled (with the top expertise in health)—and I did not know that it would be that aggressive and that unpredictable, to kill hundreds of thousands in the USA and more than one million in the world so far. And I did not know that health care professionals would feel so helpless and hopeless.

As the news of people dying by the thousands in such a short time went around the world, fear started to mount in people's minds and hearts, and the alarming daily news became a plague itself, making people panic from fear of COVID-19. But those who fear the Lord run to Him in such a time like this, to find refuge and to be safe—because the name of the Lord is a fortified tower, as is written in Proverbs 18:10. "The name of the Lord is a fortified tower; the righteous run to it and are safe" (Proverbs 18:10 NIV). That is because in God is love, and in love there is no fear. "For God gave us a spirit not of fear but of power and love and self-control" (2 Timothy 1:7 ESV).

Anxiety and Depression from COVID-19

"Fear not, for I am with you; be not dismayed, for I am your God. I will strengthen you, yes, I will help you, I will uphold you with My righteous right hand" (Isaiah 41:10 NKJV).

The fear of dying cripples people. Increased anxiety and depression have been noticed since COVID-19 started. Czeisler, Lane, Petrosky, et. al. demonstrated that "the coronavirus disease 2019 (COVID-19) pandemic has been associated with mental health challenges related to the morbidity and mortality caused by the disease and to mitigation activities, including the impact of physical distancing and stay-at-home orders. Symptoms of anxiety disorder and depressive disorder increased considerably in the United States during April–June of 2020, compared with the same period in 2019."[3]

Anxiety, depression, and other neurocognitive disorders were not strange to me due to my experience of more than three decades in memory care facilities, providing prolonged hours of care to residents with different kinds of dementia and increased anxiety and depression.

Fear, anxiety, and depression increased when people were advised in the beginning that if they got COVID-19 symptoms, they needed to "stay home," creating the "sicken-in-place" paradigm; and if the symptoms got worse, to call their primary care provider to let them know about the symptoms in order to be screened by phone for the COVID-19 virus and/or to call 911 to get hospitalized to get the needed treatment, creating the "hospital-dependent for COVID-19" model. It sounded like a strange model to me, knowing that for about thirty years we had provided care to people in a home-like environment in a community-based care setting to keep people out of the hospital.

CHAPTER 2

Gap in Primary Care During a Pandemic

No Early Treatment Protocol

My heart was broken for these sick patients at home, living in fear because the primary care providers were limited or even depleted of early treatment protocols and approaches to intervene appropriately to help out-patients, beyond over-the-counter medication (OTC) and herbal preparations and/or home remedies. People were waiting too long to get interventions on time and started to develop pneumonia—which in many cases, when the patients had other co-morbidities, was difficult to treat empirically at home. The fear increased with every symptom worsening.

Medical providers in hospitals learned from their own experience to treat the severe, acute symptoms based on the pathophysiology caused by the COVID-19 virus. Only in a primary care setting were we relaxed, being encouraged to tell patients to care for themselves at home with over-the-counter (OTC) preparations and home remedies until symptoms got worse, and then to go to the hospital. As primary care providers, we could have learned from hospital interventions that could have been started earlier, at home, to prevent hospitalization and death. At this point I despaired for those suffering with multiple COVID-19 symptoms. I could give them nothing but God's promise: "Fear not, for I am with you; be not dismayed, for I am your God. I will strengthen you, yes, I will help you, I will uphold you with My righteous right hand" (Isaiah 41:10 NKJV).

Putting our trust in God and rejoicing in the fact that He is our help in time of need and our Protector, and is holding us with His mighty hand and giving us strength in this terrible pandemic time, is extremely important for our physical and spiritual health. Sadness and depression deepen the sickness in our body, affecting all systems down to the bones—drying them up, depleting our body of energy and strength, as is written in Proverbs 17:12. "A cheerful heart is good medicine, but a crushed spirit dries up the bones" (Proverbs 17:22 NIV). We became a nation with a crushed spirit, with no solutions for interventions except God's mercy.

"Sicken-in-Place" Paradigm

A lack of randomized, controlled clinical studies and scientific information led to a lack of guidance and protocols for early interventions in primary care settings, for providers to provide medical care based on the best evidence for outpatients with COVID-19. That left general practitioners in primary care practice without solutions to treat COVID-19 patients and to alleviate the fear and prevent panic attacks that affected more— their immunity and their health conditions, leading to more frightening symptoms and increased fear of death. The absence of randomized controlled studies created a gap in primary care and a "sicken-in-place" paradigm.

I started to receive calls myself from very sick people in our community—hearing their weak voices, exhausted from COVID-19 symptoms and panicking on the phone—who were afraid to call their provider because they were so sick that they would be sent to the ER and be hospitalized. They were very afraid of the hospital due to the need for ventilator therapy and were afraid of a bad outcome. Many patients reported that they had heard on the news and social media that hospitals were full with patients with COVID-19, and that some people died after they were placed on a ventilator. I could hear the agony in their voices when they called me, begging for treatment for their symptoms with an unpredictable outcome, and my heart was aching with the pain of each sick person and each call that I received from them.

Determined to Find Solutions

I was determined to help those patients suffering from the terrible symptoms of COVID-19, and I started to look for any study that would address early interventions at home, to find solutions for our suffering patients. A statement found in a study that was published in a medical journal with a good reputation—The American Journal of Medicine—on 7 August 2020 recognized that "Approximately nine months of the severe acute respiratory syndrome coronavirus 2 (SARS-CoV-2 [COVID-19]) spreading across the globe has led to widespread COVID-19 acute hospitalizations and death. The rapidity and highly communicable nature of the SARS-CoV-2 outbreak has hampered the design and execution of definitive randomized controlled trials of therapy outside of the clinic or hospital." That is alarming, and very scary for a general practitioner in primary care management facing an inability to intervene during a crisis to save lives.

Dr. Peter A. McCullough et. al. discuss in this article the importance of outpatient treatment based on the COVID-19 infection's pathophysiology in the absence of randomized controlled trials as scientific evidence to prevent hospitalization and death from COVID-19. He stated, "In the absence of clinical trial results, physicians must use what has been learned about the pathophysiology of SARS-CoV-2 infection in determining early outpatient treatment of the illness with the aim of preventing hospitalization or death."[4]

Professional people in hospitals learned quickly about the disease caused by the COVID-19 infection's pathophysiology, as they were exposed to so many severe cases and had developed protocols based on the information they had gathered throughout this time about the advanced pathophysiology caused by the virus in hospital settings. But some people continued to die because they got to the hospital too late, when the symptoms got worse and damage to the lungs and other organs had started to happen already from the inflammatory process caused by the COVID-19 virus. It started to aggressively multiply in the lungs and the entire body while the patient was waiting at home due to "sicken-in-place" recommendations, which allowed for the symptoms to get worse, which could have been prevented with early interventions by primary care at home.

CHAPTER 3

Hypervigilant Actions

The "Battle" and the Struggle to Prevent Disaster

The struggle throughout the entire world was evident: the uncertainty about the origin of the virus and the mechanism of spreading it throughout the entire world, and the lack of expertise in knowing the COVID-19 infection's pathophysiology in order to treat the disease caused by this aggressive virus in a segment of population with other underlying conditions. We were just one month from the beginning of the year 2020, and on January 31, 2020, entry to the USA was banned and the proclamation was issued to prevent risk of further transmission of the virus and to prevent further disaster in the USA.[5]

Top leaders in our country at that time criticized the President for being so prudent in taking actions to keep Americans safe from a vicious virus that could kill millions if no prudency was applied. The media created such great tension in the USA population by spreading the news against the President's prudent actions, leading to more struggles with the fear of the pandemic. Stephen Strang stated in his book God, Trump, and COVID-19: How the Pandemic Is Affecting Christians, the World, and America's 2020 Election: "At the time, there was sharp criticism from Democrats, most notably Joe Biden, who condemned 'Trump's record of hysteria, xenophobia, and fear-mongering' after he announced the China travel restrictions. Trump said Democrats 'loudly criticized and protested' his travel restrictions and that Biden 'called me a racist' because of the decision. Trump may have slightly overstated the Democratic opposition's position. But according to The Hill, on January 31, 2020, Speaker of the House Nancy Pelosi said President Trump's decision to extend the travel ban to six African nations was 'outrageous, un-American and threatened the rule of law.' That statement didn't age well. In addition, the World Health Organization (WHO) tweeted on January 14 that there was no clear evidence of human-to-human transmission of the virus, but by January 23 the organization said human-to-human transmission was occurring."[6] Then, several weeks after that: "The World Health Organization (WHO) on March 11, 2020, has declared the novel coronavirus (COVID-19) outbreak a global pandemic."[7]

The battle with incertitude and unpredictability continues even today in managing this "invisible enemy," and the struggles continue in proving what works and what does not work, scientifically, in the absence of scientific results of randomized clinical studies. In the beginning, like the majority of general practitioners in the primary care setting, I was relaxed, abiding by the rules and regulations to "Stay Home to Save Lives." Practicing telemedicine from my office at home, I told patients that if they got sick from COVID-19 (promoting the "sicken-in-place" paradigm for our patients) and their symptoms got worse, to call first the emergency department to be triaged by well-trained staff for presumptive COVID-19 symptoms, and if needed, to call 911 to be evaluated by professional people per protocol if they had COVID-19 symptoms. The 911 staff needed to know that they were presenting with CO-VID-19 symptoms in order to use personal protective equipment (PPE), per protocol, and extra precautions for everyone's safety.

Panic and Desperation

But news started to spread rapidly about acquaintances and close family friends being sick, in our community and abroad, and being admitted to the hospital and placed on ventilators for as long as two to three weeks, causing long-term damage to the lungs and other organs. A few of our relatives in Europe and some close friends were affected by COVID-19 and passed away in a very short time, leaving their families (our relatives) with deep emotional pain and psychological trauma. Early in the spring, I got news from close family relatives that one aunt, one brother-in-law's cousin, one niece's brother-in-law, and three close friends between fifty and eighty years of age had passed away in a very short time period. That was alarming news for me that this virus was aggressive and unpredictable, and that anyone could become a victim at any time. Then I received calls from our community here in the USA that some of our friends were very sick in the hospital and on a ventilator, and three well-known persons in our community passed away.

In their desperation and terrible distress, people started to call me, asking about the treatments available and what they could do to escape the bad news dissemination by the media that early intervention was "misinformation" by frontline doctors in primary care. Patients started to panic when they were left with the uncomfortable "sicken-in-place" approach by primary care and were pressed to look for solutions in other countries. I realized that many patients from minority groups were treating themselves at home with medications from foreign countries. Many patients told me that they had started to take medications as soon as they felt sick, and they texted me pictures with medications from foreign countries, and I realized that many of them were bringing medications from outside of the USA. Many had medications from Europe, Italy, Russia, Romania, Canada, and Mexico. I heard that some of them had brought medications even from Africa. People were afraid of death from COVID-19, as the media emphasized the subject and disseminated information about the numbers of deaths rising rapidly. Many patients took the matter into their own hands to save their lives, bypassing primary care settings. Fear of the COVID-19 pandemic made people self-medicate in spite of our medical emphasis to NOT TAKE any medication without medical advice from a health care provider.

In my thoughts, I had the outrageous question: *How that can be possible in the most developed country with the highest civilization and the most qualified experts in the world?* American citizens needed to struggle and to live in desperation to get to the point of seeking help and bringing medications from undeveloped countries. My instinct told me that something was not right in medicine during this pandemic, when patients were presented with no solutions during the most stressful time of their lives from medicine and primary care practices where they are supposed to get their first intervention for their wellbeing and to prevent hospitalization.

Escaping for Their Lives

People turned to telemedicine online to find treatments and solutions from pharmacies in other states and other countries, because the majority of pharmacies were not allowed to honor doctors' orders and prescriptions to provide "off label" treatment in the most needed time. It must have been their instincts telling them that they must "run to the mountains"—in their case, to a different state or foreign country, as I described above—to get medication so the virus would not destroy them. As the Word of God gives instructions to the people He wanted to save in Genesis: "So it came to pass, when they had brought them outside, that he said, 'Escape for your life! Do not look behind you nor stay anywhere in the plain. Escape to the mountains, lest you be destroyed'" (Genesis 19:17 NKJV).

Another scripture came to mind when I was reflecting on people's actions in their desperate situations, seeking wisdom from God to escape death from COVID-19 by seeking solutions from other resources—and even other countries—to be able to treat themselves and their families, in order to escape the symptoms created by the virus and the fear of dying from COVID-19. The ancient people who feared the LORD experienced supernatural power and divine protection and divine intervention in their lives, as in Exodus 1:15-21, saving the lives of the new baby boys during the pandemic created by Pharaoh, Egypt's leader. "The king of Egypt said to the Hebrew midwives, whose names were Shiphrah and Puah, 'When you are helping the Hebrew women during childbirth on the delivery stool, if you see that the baby is a boy, kill him; but if it is a girl, let her live.' The midwives, however, feared God and did not do what the king of Egypt had told them to do; they let the boys live. Then the king of Egypt summoned the midwives and asked them, 'Why have you done this? Why have you let the boys live?' The midwives answered Pharaoh, 'Hebrew women are not like Egyptian women; they are vigorous and give birth before the midwives arrive.' So God was kind to the midwives and the people increased and became even more numerous. And because the midwives feared God, he gave them families of their own" (Exodus 1:15-21 NIV). I realized that history repeats itself, and that people who were super vigilant and treated themselves before arriving at the primary care office or ER did not die from the virus infection.

Many patients stated that they went through the "valley of the shadow of death." One particular patient, R (dear to our family), confessed: "I have seen death last night with my own eyes" when symptoms from COVID-19 got worse at home without early intervention from primary care practitioners. I cannot imagine how stressful and fearful it must be to be close to dying and to be alert, all the time knowing that you could die at any moment. One patient, who was very sick from the virus, stated that he felt "like dying" during the night and like he "would not last until morning." But he prayed and trusted the LORD through all the pain and suffering, and He spared my patient's life. Psalm 23 came many times into my head when I heard patients going through "the valley of the shadow of death."

"Though I walk through the valley of the shadow of death, I will fear no evil: for thou art with me" (Psalm 23:4 KJV). That was the only hope I could give in that moment. You can entice the patient to go to the hospital, but each patient wanted to prevent hospitalization.

In those conditions, you want to do whatever it takes to save someone's life. We are thinking about the highest authority to guide us in making decisions on how to treat those patients going through the fear of death. I did look up to the Highest Authority, who made me feel those patients' pain during the darkest moment of their life and guided me to make decisions to help them in their most critical moment, with the best of medicine and the best of Christ.

CHAPTER 4

Kindness, Love, and Compassion During a Pandemic

"And now may the LORD show kindness and truth to you. I also will repay you this kindness, because you have done this thing" (2 Samuel 2:6 NKJV).

Showing Kindness

Early in the pandemic, almost all pharmacies said that they could not fill prescriptions for HCQ for patients with COVID-19, because they did not have enough supplies for their patients who have used this medication for years for rheumatoid arthritis (RA), lupus, and other conditions (if they filled the prescriptions for people with COVID-19). That raised a question in my mind: whether we could be kind and give ten tablets of HCQ as a treatment for five days to a distressed person with viral symptoms suffering from the virus, along with other medications to prevent hospitalization, when other patients with RA or lupus take about 730 tablets per year and about 7, 300 tablets in ten years. Could these patients, who take this medication for so many years, use different alternatives to address their conditions, prescribed by rheumatologists who now have more options then HCQ to treat RA, lupus, etc.? When you are kind to other people you receive a great reward, as is written in 2 Samuel 2:6. "And now may the LORD show kindness and truth to you. I also will repay you this kindness, because you have done this thing" (2 Samuel 2:6 NKJV).

Even though we do not share the same vision in our practice, medicine, expertise, profession, or politics, when so many people's lives are badly affected by the virus we must act with kindness, even if it is to our enemy. "But love your enemies, do good, and lend, hoping for nothing in return; and your reward will be great, and you will be sons of the Most High. For He is kind to the unthankful and evil" (Luke 6:35 NKJV). When the President of the USA was willing to share publicly and was not ashamed to tell the world that he was taking an anti-malaria drug to prevent COVID-19, we all needed to rejoice and embrace that solution (not criticize), until we had scientific data to prove what works and what does not work. "Rejoice and be exceedingly glad, for great is your reward in heaven, for so they persecuted the prophets who were before you" (Matthew 5:12 NKJV) But instead of rejoicing over the President's statement, the "experts" were outrageous, starting a "war" against this solution on every channel and on social media, putting the entire population in terrible distress of the unknown "invisible enemy" COVID-19 without a solution, when there was a solution.

Here is what Dr. Naomi Florea Buda, Associate Professor and Vice Chair, University of Southern California, wrote and cited Peter McCullough, MD, who emphasized, "'When the history of COVID-19 is written,' McCullough said, 'it will be "very unkind" to those who crafted a paradigm that withheld treatment until patients were so debilitated that hospitalization was needed.'" [8]

The algorithm in the article "Pathophysiological Basis and Rationale for Early Outpatient Treatment of SARS-CoV-2 (COVID-19) Infection," by et. al., published in The American Journal of Medicine (available online, 7 August 2020), talks about the necessity of early interventions for COVID-19 patients to prevent hospitalization. A low dose of well-known hydroxychloroquine is recommended in the algorithm with other well-known medications to treat early COVID-19 symptoms for outpatients' early management.

Love Casts Out Fear, Even in Medicine

"There is no fear in love; but perfect love casts out fear, because fear involves torment. But he who fears has not been made perfect in love. We love Him because He first loved us" (1 John 4:18-20 NKJV).

When the news was spreading in the first months that people were dying by the thousands daily in other countries, fear gripped people's hearts when watching the news. I knew what that implied. I have spent about three decades providing end-of-life care to dying people in long-term settings. I have seen thousands of dying patients during my experience in providing palliative care at bedside to sick people in their last days of life on this planet. I know very well what the dying process looks like and the devastating emotions of anxiety, depression, and despair caused by death. Patients are suffering, families are in desperation, and professional people are helpless and hopeless in front of death. Everybody is devastated by the dying process, especially when it is as unexpected as it is from COVID-19.

It was August 20, 2020 when I received a call from one of my family members (I call her Li), stating that one of her residents in a memory care facility, where she is the executive director and the registered nurse of house, had tested positive for COVID-19. Because she spent extended hours (twelve to fourteen hours every day) in the facility, she needed to have her test done, but the results would come back only in four to eight days (because there were no rapid tests available at that time) and she needed to isolate herself. She experienced no symptoms in the beginning when she was tested but some general fatigue and a dry cough occasionally. She asked me what she could do to be able to continue to work, because she "could not afford to abandon the residents" in that memory care facility and stay home in quarantine.

She was in the facility for prolonged hours during the pandemic to make sure that staff and residents were taken care of and safe. I knew her heart for those frail people who were exposed to the cruel virus. She loved her patients. During the pandemic time she worked constantly, with no days off the entire time, caring for the most vulnerable population. Her love was stronger than her fear of COVID-19. Her faith moved mountains every day. She lived out God's Word, as written in 1 John 4:18-20: "There is no fear in love; but perfect love casts out fear, because fear involves torment. But he who fears has not been made perfect in love. We love Him because He first loved us" (1 John 4:18-20 NKJV).

Big Concerns Touched My Heart

I knew exactly where Li came from with her big concerns. Her kindness, love, and compassion for the frail, disabled elderly touched my heart. I had provided care to the elderly with multiple chronic conditions and neurocognitive disorders who were totally dependent in all activities of daily living (ADLs), and I knew how much work was required in a memory care facility in order to meet the needs of all the residents with so many disabilities and to provide support for the entire staff and families.

I had to come up with a solution to help Li get through this pandemic period, when more residents were testing positive with mild symptoms but which could become a catastrophe if the executive director and RN and staff had to stay in quarantine at home. It happened in some community-based facilities and nursing homes, when patients got very sick from COVID-19 and their caregivers tested positive too, that they needed to quarantine themselves per the rules (even if no symptoms were present), so they quit coming to work in the most crucial time. They had to be moved to other facilities, causing more trauma to these fragile and frail residents already in critical condition. Li preferred to be "isolated at work to be able to provide care for the sick" (because her symptoms were mild). She wanted to sequestrate the symptoms in her body to stop them at any price in order to not get sicker, and to be able to continue to provide care to the residents in the memory care at any cost to meet the residents' needs during the pandemic time when family members or visitors were not allowed in the facility.

Based on her clinical presentation, she was functioning as normal except for feeling a little tired and coughing occasionally at that time. All other caregivers and staff were exposed to that case of COVID-19 but were not symptomatic. They had been the same team and the same residents for the last several months, like a big family (being in their own bubble). All of the staff and the residents had been tested for COVID-19, but no results were available yet. All staff respected all of the CDC recommendations and had all PPE in place to protect themselves and the residents. My mind was spinning, knowing what could happen with all the news about the unpredictable progression of the disease caused by the COVID-19 virus—hospitalization, and in some cases, death.

Li's big concern touched my heart, and in my desperation to help her, I was looking for information about the treatments available for outpatient clinics and options for treatment in patients who were exposed to the virus and who developed mild-to-moderate symptoms, to further help Li who was in desperation at that time for medical intervention.

COVID-19 AND POST COVID-19 ALLEVIATE THE FEAR

Compelled by Compassion

"Why are we sitting here until we die?" (2 Kings 7:3 NKJV).

During the pandemic, with the "Stay Home/Save Lives" condition we had to treat all kinds of diseases, based on clinical presentation, by telemedicine. My question (with a burning desire to see patients healed) during this time was, why could we not treat symptoms of patients with COVID-19 earlier at home (as I described above) to prevent hospitalization and premature death?

One of the patients who was struggling with COVID-19 asked me, "Why in the primary care setting are general practitioners and providers so relaxed and not prescribing medications to treat the symptoms of COVID-19 patients at home?" That stirred compassion in my heart and made me think more about why, during this pandemic, we were waiting for people to get sick enough with severe symptoms—deteriorating before our own eyes—in order for them to go to the emergency room, terrified that they would be admitted to the hospital for more aggressive interventions that may work or not and that they would end up with post COVID-19 damage. (I will address that later.) Why could we not start that treatment earlier and prevent all of the unnecessary turmoil that patients had to go through?

I knew that the primary care setting lacked guidance to manage early COVID-19 patients to prevent hospitalization with consumption of resources, and to prevent premature death, because of the lack of randomized controlled trials. Those need several years to be achieved, but during a pandemic when we do not have much time and time is precious, to save lives we could use our common sense and experience in the medical field.

God speaks through His Word when we listen. As I was contemplating this terrible situation where we were in primary care management, the Holy Spirit brought the story to my mind that was written in God's Word about four leprous men who realized that if they did nothing during the time of crisis, they would die if they were sitting doing nothing there, or if they went into the city. But God spared their lives because they decided to move to "do something" about the situation, as written in 2 Kings 7:3-4. "Now there were four leprous men at the entrance of the gate; and they said to one another, 'Why are we sitting here until we die? If we say, "We will enter the city," the famine is in the city, and we shall die there. And if we sit here, we die also. Now therefore, come, let us surrender to the army of the Syrians. If they keep us alive, we shall live; and if they kill us, we shall only die.' And they rose at twilight to go to the camp of the Syrians; and when they had come to the outskirts of the Syrian camp, to their surprise no one was there. For the Lord had caused the army of the Syrians to hear the noise of chariots and the noise of horses—the noise of a great army; so they said to one another, 'Look, the king of Israel has hired against us the kings of the Hittites and the kings of the Egyptians to attack us!' Therefore they arose and fled at twilight, and left the camp intact—their tents, their horses, and their donkeys—and they fled for their lives" (2 Kings 7:3-7 NKJV).

I asked myself the same question: Why am I relaxed in primary care, "doing nothing" for our suffering patients with coronavirus? If I do not treat them, "they will die." It is better to treat them early, before their developed symptoms get worse, so they will not need hospitalization.

Hearing that many people during an outbreak in our community had contracted the virus so fast and were acutely developing severe symptoms and dying in a matter of weeks, my heart was filled with compassion for them. My thoughts in my mind went to King Jesus, the Son of God, who was moved with compassion when the multitudes were weary, without hope and support. "But when He saw the multitudes, He was moved with compassion for them, because they were weary and scattered, like sheep having no shepherd" (Matthew 9:36 NKJV). That verse gave me tears, because our patients infected with the COVID-19 virus were weary and with no hope. If we are in the healing field, why are our hearts not moved with compassion anymore in primary care settings?

After being moved deeply by the Holy Spirit, through the powerful Word of God, staying relaxed in the primary care setting and waiting for people to get sick with their symptoms getting worse made me so uncomfortable as a primary care provider with a mission to help the most vulnerable people with the love of Christ and with all our intellectual and material resources.

Prevent Hospitalization

"Sicken-in-Place" and "Hospital-Dependent" NOT the Right Approach

I knew that we were told to "stay home," and if we were very sick to call the emergency room's staff or go to the hospital if symptoms got worse, such as: increased breathing difficulties; persistent, severe chest pain and chest pressure; confusion; severe fatigue; weakness to the point that you cannot get up to go to the bathroom or are not able to wake up or stay awake; and if you had bluish lips and bluish face or unusual symptoms, etc. Li did not have those symptoms and could not stay home to wait for her symptoms to get worse and to have to go to the hospital. A battle in my mind was real with the "sicken-in-place" and "hospital-dependent" approach. I knew that "sicken-in-place" and "hospital-dependent" were not the right approach. Being around the sick and providing care to dying people gave me insight and made my instinct hypervigilant around sick people.

As a general practitioner, I could not stay relaxed anymore to tell people to practice "sicken-in-place" methods until they needed hospitalization. I started to look for solutions. I did look for updated information on the internet, and I did consult with experts in infectious diseases and professional people involved directly in COVID-19 patients' care in our nation and abroad, and I asked for recommendations for treatment for outpatient care for patients with COVID-19 symptoms. I realized at that time that after almost six months in this pandemic situation, with the most advanced technology in medicine and the best experts in the sciences of medicine, epidemiology, virology, pharmacy, etc., we struggled with no guidance in primary care to help people suffering with this sickness from so unpredictable and aggressive a virus as COVID-19, that kills the most vulnerable population. I realized how limited we were in the face of this so-rightly named "invisible enemy" that had created panic and physical, social, economic, and psychological disaster on entire planet.

At this point I listened to my instinct (the small voice inside of me that in many difficult situations has guided me to the right solution) and common sense to treat Li, who was battling this cruel enemy of the body, soul, and spirit, to further prevent a disastrous event from this unpredictable virus. I reviewed thoroughly the information with the protocol and the algorithm published in the *Journal of American Medicine* to make a well-informed decision, not knowing that down the road an outbreak of COVID-19 was waiting to attack our community, with more relatives and friends who needed my help as a general practitioner and primary care provider to intervene early and prevent diseases and prevent hospitalizations and premature deaths.

Early Interventions—Choose Life Solution

"I call heaven and earth as witnesses today against you, that I have set before you life and death, blessing and cursing; therefore choose life, that both you and your descendants may live" (Deuteronomy 30:19 NKJV).

Early in my education for primary care management, I liked "health promotion and disease prevention" the most, and I paid very close attention to those courses to learn more of what can be done in our society to prevent disease and promote health. I felt that health promotion and disease prevention "got into my blood" and became a part of who I am, and I wanted to do everything possible to help others understand that prevention is the key to a healthy life, physically and spiritually. (I did address that subject in my first book, *Find Your Peace*.)

When diseases from the COVID-19 virus started, I was worried that nothing had been discovered for early interventions for outpatient treatment to prevent hospitalization except over-the-counter medication for low-grade fever, mild to moderate pain, and for cough to some extent. Learning that COVID-19 was so unpredictable and extremely aggressive in those who become infected with a higher viral load, I knew that we needed to also be aggressive with our early medical interventions and expertise to prevent further damage to the body, and that OTC would not be enough to treat our patients in desperate need of severe acute respiratory syndrome coronavirus 2 (SARS-CoV-2) medical care.

All of the media reports were only on hospitals' interventions, as experts were learning about the pathophysiology of the diseases caused by COVID-19. My heart was sinking when we were left with no solutions in the primary care setting for early interventions for patients in the community who were infected with the virus and were afraid to go to the emergency room, being afraid of hospitalization. Many of them were thinking that once in the hospital they would be placed on a ventilator and die. A close friend—I call her Mia—from our community who was an active businesswoman and was exposed to the COVID-19 virus, stayed home per medical advice; the symptoms got worse in the second week of infection, and when she went to the hospital she was told, "You came too late," and she died in the hospital at age fifty-five. That shook the entire community to the core with great fear of the COVID-19 virus.

I heard that concern over and over again from patients, their hearts gripped with intense fear and panic. Many patients stated that they had heard reports that thousands of people had died in the hospital in different parts of the USA (NY) and different parts of the world (Italy and Brazil) in a very short time during this pandemic. The majority of those who were dying were placed on a ventilator as the last resort and never recovered. Each patient who tested positive or developed symptoms when exposed to the virus begged me to help him/her to get treatment at home for early signs and symptoms of the COVID-19 virus, to prevent hospitalization.

That raised a concerned question in my mind: Why could we not treat COVID-19 patients at home earlier instead, as the symptoms began? This would prevent panic from fear of the hospital, and so much psychological distress caused by untreated symptoms and by thoughts of uncertainty and the unknown. We could then send to the hospital only patients with severe symptoms that could not be treated at home, for close supervision and further complex interventions.

Doctors and specialists who were working with patients with COVID-19 in the hospital were also terrified by the lack of solutions to save lives. But they realized that they could treat symptoms caused by the COVID-19 virus based on the pathophysiological response of every system in the body. Many doctors and specialists posted video clips on social media, circulating useful information about what they had learned during the disease process about the pathophysiology and how they had intervened, based on their knowledge gained over the years about potential medication to save patients' lives.

Hospitalists used well-known medications from their accumulated experience of years of daily practice in medicine. Medications used before for different diseases were used now for symptoms of COVID-19 to reduce inoculation, with antiviral therapy and immuno-modulators to treat the inflammation and microthrombosis produced by the debris from inflammation from the "cytokine storm" caused by the virus. They began to administer bronchodilators via inhalers or nebulizers, and oxygen supplementation to treat breathing difficulties and the oxygen deficiency known as hypoxia, a condition caused by low oxygen levels, to assist people to breathe better.

Care at Home—Save Lives

I was very familiar with "care at home" from working in the long-term care field, because I had to provide care to acutely and chronically ill people "at home" all the time to keep those patients out of the hospital. Professional people had been talking about treatment in the home for decades, and "house calls" and "home health" were developed in order to provide care to people in the comfort of their own homes, to prevent hospitalization. Many times, we had to provide post-op care with complex interventions for patients at home using well-known, complex medications and procedures such as nebulizers and oxygen supplementation for COPD, asthma, and other lung conditions. I was familiar with caring for tracheostomies, colostomies, and ileostomies; using portable ventilators, using complex medications via nasal tubes, catheter care; and treatments for multiple chronic conditions with different kinds of medications such as antibiotics, antivirals, anti-coagulants, anti-hypertensives, anti-diabetes, and complex pain control measures, etc.

My experience of thirty years of working in long-term care facilities with a "home like" environment (as a provider, a manager, and an owner of those facilities, with residents with multiple chronic conditions treated chronically in the past with all of the medications that are used now for patients with symptoms from diseases caused by the COVID-19 virus in the hospital, except treatment via IV infusion) opened my eyes to the possibility of treating patients in the community with symptoms from COVID-19 early, in the comfort of their homes. For example: antibiotics used for upper and lower respiratory infections; anti-inflammatory drugs and steroids used for patients with inflammation in their lungs causing wheezing and difficulty breathing; immunomodulatory drugs such as hydroxychloroquine, used for about sixty years for autoimmune diseases with inflammatory processes; bronchodilators for shortness of breath and oxygen supplementation for patients with low oxygen levels from hypoxia; antipyretics for high fever, analgesics for pain, cough medications for cough, etc. I was familiar with all of those medications and the procedures for administration.

I thought that it was possible to treat patients with symptoms from the COVID-19 virus at home—with antibiotics, with anti-viral and anti-inflammatory properties, immuno-modulators and anti-inflammatory meds, bronchodilators, inhalers, nebulizers, oxygen supplementation, etc.—to treat acute, mild, and moderate symptoms in COVID-19 patients with early interventions to prevent hospitalization. That would alleviate the fear factor in those suffering patients which affects the immune system in a negative way, aggravating the symptoms from infection, leading to more decline of the patients' condition and hospitalization and premature death.

CHAPTER 6

Holy Spirit at Work

Ask, Seek, and Knock

Another verse from the Bible came to my mind that made me uncomfortable again about "doing nothing" for the suffering people in our community and that made me seek information for yearly interventions in primary care for COVID-19 patients. That verse is written in Matthew 7:7-12. "Ask, and it will be given to you; seek, and you will find; knock, and it will be opened to you. For everyone who asks receives, and he who seeks finds, and to him who knocks it will be opened. Or what man is there among you who, if his son asks for bread, will give him a stone? Or if he asks for a fish, will he give him a serpent? If you then, being evil, know how to give good gifts to your children, how much more will your Father who is in heaven give good things to those who ask Him! Therefore, whatever you want men to do to you, do also to them, for this is the Law and the Prophets" (Matthew 7:7-12 NKJV).

The Holy Spirit was working on my heart and mind to ask, seek, and knock. Compelled by compassion, I decided not to "sit here anymore" and "do nothing," and I did reach out to Dr. Naomi Florea Buda, Pharm D., Founder, Chief Pharmacy Officer, Associate Professor of Clinical Pharmacy, Vice Chair of Innovation, Chair, at University of South California Department of Experiential and Continuing Education, and Associate Professor, Infectious Diseases at Loma Linda University, to find out her thoughts on this pandemic time and what were my options for early interventions for patients with COVID-19 at a small clinic in Portland. Then I did check her professional postings on social media, and I realized that she is well informed and on top of the issues regarding treatments available for COVID-19 that are scientifically proven.

Through personal contact, she referred me to the algorithm from a study published in The American Journal of Medicine on 7 August 2020, and my eyes were opened wide and I knew that was the solution and that there was hope for patients with COVID-19 in our community. and had created the following algorithm for early intervention and treatment at home for COVID-19 patients to be provided by primary care to prevent hospitalization, and it appeared in the article "Pathophysiological Basis and Rationale for Early Outpatient Treatment of SARS-CoV-2 (COVID-19) Infection" published in The American Journal of Medicine on 7 August 2020. But the information about the algorithm was not disseminated, so we had to struggle with lack of guidance and no solutions.

The Algorithm that Saved Lives

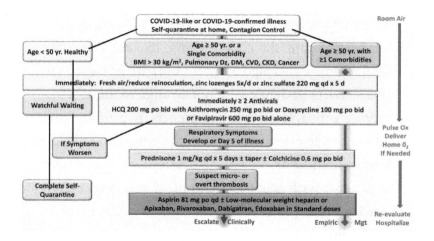

Figure 1. Treatment algorithm for COVID-19-like and confirmed COVID-19 illness in ambulatory patients at home in self-quarantine. BMI = body mass index; CKD = chronic kidney disease; CVD = cardiovascular disease; DM = diabetes mellitus; Dz = disease; HCQ = hydroxychloroquine; Mgt = management; O2 = oxygen; Ox = oximetry; Yr = year[9]

My struggle was with the rules and regulations of the FDA that as providers we must follow, but I learned quickly that "The FDA also acknowledges that physicians have the legal right to prescribe already-approved drugs 'off label' as they deem appropriate."[10]

Led by the Holy Spirit, without delay I started the treatment of symptoms for COVID-19 patients who started to call every day at the clinic during an outbreak season as an outpatient approach, based on the research done by top doctors, based on their experience in medicine and their algorithms, to save lives. The medications in this algorithm for outpatient treatment for COVID-19 patients were not strange to me as a primary care provider with experience in primary care and long-term care settings with patients with multiple chronic conditions. Those medications had been used for patients with acute and chronic diseases on a daily basis for many years. In our foster homes and memory care facilities we had administered all those medications for all those years of providing care to people with different illnesses, with no serious side effects or adverse reactions. Li called me the third day of the treatment she started for the COVID-19 virus and stated, "I cannot believe what a difference these medications have made for me. I feel like a completely different person. My energy level came back. It is a night-and-day difference."

I have witnessed firsthand the fear, anxiety, and anguish of people who have tested positive for COVID-19 and are experiencing mild, moderate, and some severe signs and symptoms that put a mark on their emotional and physical well-being, and I couldn't stay relaxed, "doing nothing" and letting people suffer with no early interventions, when we had medications available at an affordable price for everybody to treat their symptoms at home. When patients called me, I felt their emotional pain literally, and I treated every single person as a member of my own family with great responsibility, love, and compassion.

Medical Approach for Outpatients

I looked intentionally with great interest for published articles in medical journals during the pandemic, knowing that we lacked the best evidence such as randomized controlled studies that are imperative to use and the best evidence practice in caring for people with illnesses from COVID-19. But due to the short time to get the results from randomized controlled studies and to get the data on time that would guide our practice, I considered that it was imperative to use the knowledge about medications that I had accumulated over the years to treat patients early at home to prevent hospitalization, resources consumption, and premature death. et. al. emphasized in the article "Pathophysiological

Basis and Rationale for Early Outpatient Treatment of SARS-CoV-2 (COVID-19) Infection" that "Therapeutic approaches based on these principles include 1) reduction of reinoculation, 2) combination antiviral therapy, 3) immunomodulation, 4) antiplatelet/antithrombotic therapy, and 5) administration of oxygen, monitoring, and telemedicine."[11]

CHAPTER 7

Listen to the President's Heart

Learn from the President

I am reflecting on the former President's statement about the possibility of preventative actions and early interventions with HCQ, and I cannot wrap my mind around the unkind decisions to withhold treatments and interventions, waiting for patients to get so sick and debilitated by the virus that they needed hospitalization. We could have learned from the President's experience with prophylactic treatment and the frontline doctors with so much expertise in primary care management in treating these people and so many others like them earlier, to prevent hospitalization and further damage done by this virus physically, emotionally, socially, and economically, affecting people's quality of life and premature death.

I heard in March that President Trump had then stated that he was taking hydroxychloroquine prophylactically as a preventative measure. My common sense told me that the President of the USA's doctors must be the best doctors in the world. They would never prescribe unsafe medications for the President of the USA. I had prescribed low doses of hydroxychloroquine for several years for patients with rheumatoid arthritis (with other multiple chronic diseases) and lupus, and none of them reported any side effects. One particular patient with multiple chronic diseases such as diabetes, hypertension, and coronary artery disease took this medication every day for more than ten years and did not report any side effects or adverse reactions during this entire time. She even stated, "I feel good."

I knew that this medication was safe and very cheap to treat patients with diseases from COVID-19. I also knew that this medication was used by millions around the world to treat symptoms from viruses on a regular basis, and even as an over-the-counter medication for several years. But for COVID-19 symptoms, for early intervention the protocol is for a low dose of HCQ only for five days, twice a day, so a total of ten tablets (in some cases can be repeated for five more days), compared with those patients taking thousands of tablets of HCQ during those ten to twenty years for RA, lupus, and malaria.

It Worked for Him—Saved His Life

During the pandemic, the President recognized that there were no randomized controlled trials and scientific evidence to prove the effectiveness of hydroxychloroquine. "We know that there is no scientific evidence, but it has worked with me," he claimed. And he was right, because during a pandemic time there is no time to get the results from a randomized controlled trial for the best evidence practice.

The President was criticized for speaking publicly about taking this medication prophylactically. It was negatively reported that "hydroxychloroquine was first touted by Mr. Trump in March. Two months later he surprised journalists by saying he had begun taking the unproven medication to ward off the virus" when hydroxychloroquine is a safe medication, used for more than five decades by millions of people. That lie was a big disservice to the USA's population, criticizing the President for his prudent measure to save his life during a pandemic time, when there was no time for randomized controlled studies results to be available for such an aggressive virus that had killed hundreds of thousands. They made an untrue statement that the medication was unproven. The medication was a well-tested medication and used by millions around the globe for more than five decades. It was used as an "off label" medication, like many other drugs used in medicine by medical professionals all the time to treat symptoms from illnesses caused by viruses, bacteria, and other different diseases in the body. The President used the best information we had in medicine at that time, during a crisis created by a pandemic, prescribed for him by his medical doctors and experts in medicine. That was a clue for people to do the same to save their lives.[12]

It was reported by the BBC that as a result of the public disclosure by the President about his precautions and interventions to prevent COVID-19 symptoms, the demand for hydroxychloroquine had increased. "There's been widespread interest in hydroxychloroquine as both a preventative measure and for treating patients with coronavirus. President Trump has used it as a preventative measure, and President Bolsonaro of Brazil has also taken it."[13]

It is well known that "hydroxychloroquine has long been used to treat malaria as well as other conditions such as lupus and arthritis. It's used to reduce fever and inflammation, and the hope has been that it can also inhibit the virus that causes COVID-19."[14]

But there are many medical professional doctors with many years of experience in medicine from whom we can learn about the best approach to fighting CO-VID-19 during a pandemic time, when no scientific evidence from randomized controlled trials exists.

The President of the USA Was Right

"But He answered and said to them, 'I tell you that if these should keep silent, the stones would immediately cry out'" (Luke 19:40 NKJV).

The President of the USA did not keep silent, and he cried out to tell the American people and the world that there was hope when he disclosed to the public that he was taking HCQ and encouraged the American people—who were rightly scared by this unpredictable and aggressive virus—to take it prophylactically as he did. He was right in presenting HCQ as being the antidote for COVID-19 for the majority of the USA population if taken early, before the symptoms worsened. The American people and all media should celebrate that here in the USA we had a solution for the virus, and we had a leader who did not keep silent and was disclosing from his personal experience so many other lives could be saved.

Andrew Mark Miller wrote an article, "Study Finds 84% Fewer Hospitalizations for Patients Treated with Controversial Drug Hydroxychloroquine" in the Washington Examiner, which stated that the study, set to be published in the *International Journal of Antimicrobial Agents* in December, determined that "low-dose hydroxychloroquine combined with zinc and azithromycin was an effective therapeutic approach against

COVID-19." A total of 141 patients diagnosed with the coronavirus were treated with the three-drug cocktail over a period of five days and compared to a control group of 377 people who tested positive for the virus but were not given the treatment. The study found that "the odds of hospitalization of treated patients was 84% less than in the untreated patients," and only one patient died from the group being treated with the drugs compared to 13 deaths in the untreated group.[15]

The media silenced the President of the USA with their unkind, negative reports and criticism and left the entire population of the USA with no hope, tormented by fear. "The stones will cry out" for those who were not treated with early interventions prophylactically and who died unnecessarily.

Criticized for Saving Lives

Frontline doctors, including Simone Gold, MD, with a team of prominent physicians were speaking (on a video viewed by millions of people) about using hydroxychloroquine medication for their patients in the early phase of viral infection with great results, but they were mocked and harshly criticized for their early interventions to treat suffering people from the diseases caused by COVID-19. Through censorship, the media removed the information from their platforms, stating that they spread "misinformation." "The video was retweeted by President Donald Trump and his son, Donald Trump Jr., and spread like wildfire online, garnering millions of views before it was removed by Facebook, Twitter and YouTube for what the social media companies said was spreading misinformation about the coronavirus."[16]

That is an outrageous statement made by the media, to call "misinformation" the treatment of low-dose HCQ given for five days (ten tablets), when many states have legalized drugs such as marijuana with multiple bad consequences for the long term, leading to neurocognitive syndromes, psychosis, and anti-motivation condition in the younger population. Many become homeless and live in the most miserable conditions, in tents worse than in a third-world environment, with no water to wash hands, no bathrooms for their necessities, no shower, no laundry, no civilized conditions. I do not hear words of criticism on TV or social media platforms about all the bad consequences of legalized marijuana, especially for younger people who are destroying their future.

Brian Tyson, MD, board certified in Family Medicine with fourteen years of ER and hospital medicine experience at All Valley Urgent Care in El Centro, California, who saved about 4,500 patients suffering from Covid-19 with early interventions in his practice, wrote in The Desert Review about his speech at the US Supreme Court in Washington DC about COVID-19 early interventions to prevent hospitalization. He stated, "We can go back to school! We can go back to work! We can go back to life! We can go back to being Americans! We will not let fear take our freedom! I spoke on those steps. That was a moment I will never forget. It truly was incredible. I have always wanted to do something great for my country, knowing that my grandfathers served in WW2, Vietnam, and Korea. I thought of my grandpa Tyson. My dad served in Vietnam. How scared were they? What must it have been like to have to go into an actual war? This is my war, and it's not over. We are still fighting the fight, and we will continue to do so. I hoped the video would be a tool that other physicians could see and hear. We need everyone to see the success we had. When it was finally posted on YouTube, it was exciting—it started to go viral, and then something happened. It was taken down! Why? Why would you take down a video with the knowledge, research, links, and website, where everyone can see what we are doing? Why? I don't have any reason. I can't believe that big tech and government controls want to see people die. Why would you take down the message of hope? Why would you take down the message of treatment? Why do you want to continue living in fear, when there are clear treatment options now? There are multiple options. Peter McCullough and his peers published the first peer-reviewed pathway to outpatient treatment in the *American Journal of Medicine*, and that too was recently taken down. We had to get Senate influence to have them re-publish it! That should upset people all over the world. Think about it—the world is looking to us to find a treatment or a cure, and when we do, it gets taken down? ...I was able to get raw video, and we published it again and again. We will keep publishing it over and over, until it is recognized all over the world that we don't need to be afraid anymore. People need to know that we will survive this pandemic, just like those of the past. There is treatment available. It works when used early, and it is very effective."[17]

I could hear in Dr. Tyson's tone of voice his compassion for suffering patients to get treated early, with the best we have available in medicine. I sensed the passion in his heart for the world to instill hope in peoples' minds and to alleviate the fear of COVID-19. I also heard his great, intense agony and disappointment over the media's actions to fight against the information that would bring a ray of hope and to deprive the world of the solution that could stop the pandemic with its loss of patients' lives, leaving nations with damage economically, financially, socially, mentally, and emotionally for generations.

CHAPTER 8

The Highest Authority

God's Gifts: Science and Faith

During this "war" with a merciless virus and the "war" with outrageous negative media reports on treatments for COVID-19 and actions to intimidate hard-working practitioners trying to save people's lives, I had to turn to the Highest Authority to help me make decisions in providing care to patients suffering from life-threatening diseases caused by COVID-19. In all my decisions to treat suffering patients during this pandemic time—not only suffering from physical pain and sickness and diseases, but in great psychological distress—I needed to obey the Highest Authority, who created science and who gives faith as gift that has guided me always when I have needed direction in my life. Science and faith are both God's gifts to humanity.

While living in a communist country for about three decades, as a person of faith I gained experience in how to cope with uncertainty in a place where cruel communist leaders with no faith in God dictated to the entire nation how to live our daily lives during crises with no hope, creating more confusion and oppression when life hurt the most. When I faced difficulties and persecutions for following Christ with the highest morals in the universe, in those long years under a communist regime and dictatorship, I learned that God has the Highest Authority, and that I needed to trust God's Word and run under His mighty wings for divine protection. In every circumstance, I needed to look up at the Highest Authority that gave me direction and guidance in every step I had to take—which was the Living Word of God, that has the same sovereign power today, for every person who believes in God and for those who do not.

"From the end of the earth I will cry to You, when my heart is overwhelmed; lead me to the rock that is higher than I" (Psalm 61:2 NKJV).

Why Withholding Effective Early Treatment?

As the President wondered why we did not want to use early interventions in patients with COVID-19, so Peter A. McCullough, MD, MPH, noticed the unkindness of professional people in primary care and politicians rising above experts in medicine. Also, Mr. Stephen Strang noticed the cruelty of withholding effective early treatment in patients suffering from this aggressive, unpredictable virus in his book God, Trump, and COVID-19: How the Pandemic Is Affecting Christians, the World, and America's 2020 Election. When he addressed the hydroxychloroquine issue, he stated: "The question is, why would Democrats want to stop the flow of a possible effective treatment to their citizens? Most likely for political purposes, it seems. They just don't want to give the president a win. They even referred to the treatment as 'snake oil' even though several studies and medical journals from France, Italy, and China show promising and effective results. Meanwhile, India and other countries limited hydroxychloroquine from being sent out of their countries to other countries. President Trump eventually worked hard to construct a deal with both India and Israel to have millions of doses sent to the United States. It seems the polarization of the American political climate has hit new levels, as even in a pandemic situation there can't seem to be agreement on getting fast and effective medication help to the people."[18]

The same question echoed in my mind: "Why in primary care are we withholding early treatment and waiting for people to 'sicken-in-place,' living in fear of dying from those symptoms that are worsening as the time passes by, and causing a terrible distress physically and emotionally so that they will have no choice but hospitalization?" In my desperation to save people's lives in our community so they would not be overwhelmed with fear and despair, God gave me an experience in my practice with multiple patients experiencing signs and symptoms of COVID-19 in different stages, and I have seen firsthand their quick recovery if treatment was started early. I have also observed very slow recovery—even hospitalization with lung damage—if patients with symptoms started treatment late in the course of the illness caused by COVID-19.

CHAPTER 9

Saving Lives Experience

My Experience with Early Interventions

One morning the telephone was ringing, and I heard a weak voice at the other end stating that she had a dream that I could help her with her desperate need for treatment for terrible symptoms in her family. I was speechless, realizing how God cared for His children by moving in my heart to seek solutions for the helpless that He loves, giving them dreams about where to go for help. And after that, many other patients were led to call for early interventions for their worsening symptoms from COVID-19. Over fifty patients called with COVID-19 during a few weeks' period during that outbreak. They called for help when many providers refused to treat COVID-19 symptoms at home. Each patient with COVID-19 had a unique clinical presentation of the symptoms. But all reported at least five mild-to-moderate symptoms in the first week, such as sore throat, dry cough, shortness of breath, fever, chills, night sweats, headaches, dizziness, muscles pain, nausea, vomiting, diarrhea, lost appetite, lost taste and smell, weakness, fatigue, pink eye, etc. They reported that they had used over-the-counter preparations for fever, pain, and cough with minimum results, but the symptoms did not go away. But the longer they waited, those symptoms got worse, and patients started to experience more compulsive cough, shortness of breath, hypoxia, severe weakness, increased fatigue, dizziness, hypotension, and persistent fever, panicking as the time passed by and their health condition deteriorated due to the increased inflammation process from the cytokine storm—a reaction of their immune systems to the COVID-19 viral infection.

Worse Cases Lead to More Anxiety

The worst-case scenario was when the fever increased to over 101 degrees Fahrenheit and would not cease (after taking Tylenol and ibuprofen regularly for ten days), and the oxygen levels started to drop below 89 percent even after using an in-home nebulizer or oxygen supplementation. That was the time when a care provider needed to be on alert to monitor very closely the progression of the symptoms and the patient's decline in health condition and to send them to the hospital for more advanced and aggressive interventions.

When their oxygen levels started to drop below 89 percent, the patients coughed more and they experienced shortness of breath, showing signs of developing pneumonia that was life-threatening due to the inflammation process caused by the cytokine storm at the alveoli level. This is created by the immune system when fighting the COVID-19 virus, which further causes micro thrombosis, abnormal blood clots in the lungs' blood vessels, developing into acute respiratory distress syndrome (ARDS). These patients needed to go to the hospital right away for close monitoring and advanced interventions. But with early outpatient interventions, I helped hundreds of patients to recover at home from COVID-19 as from a "flu-like illness" but "more aggressive," like described by the patients who gave their testimony of how their symptoms improved in two to four days.

It was satisfying to see the results of early interventions in mild and moderate COVID-19 symptoms that prevented hospitalization of the patients with all its consequences. Many patients and their families got into profound psychological distress when early interventions were refused by their primary care providers. For example, one of the patients—I call him Je—who tested positive for COVID-19 stated that he went to the primary care provider, who told him to "isolate at home and to wait for my symptoms to aggravate and only then to call my doctor." In the meantime, he was told to drink tea with honey and to take Tylenol or other over-the-counter cold medications. This patient's anxiety increased so much, knowing from his close friends that the symptoms could aggravate quickly with no interventions—and they ended up in the hospital and a few of them were put on a ventilator, and some passed away.

Another patient—I call her Covey—with a compulsive cough and shortness of breath, whose oxygen saturation dropped to 90 percent overnight after eight days of mild symptoms from the virus, was told that she needed a chest X-ray first to see if she needed treatment. This patient was in desperation because there was no place to go to get the chest X-ray done. "Nobody wanted to do a chest X-ray for me," she stated, because she had tested positive for COVID-19 and needed to wait two weeks to quarantine first. She did not want to go to the ER when she was so sick. Nothing else matters when you cannot breathe. She was in day eight after the symptoms began to manifest, and they were worsening instead of getting better. She tried to treat herself with home remedies and OTC preparations, with no results. Her symptoms got worse and worse every day, and she needed empirical interventions and more aggressive interventions right away at home for pneumonia from COVID-19, (which is different from other kinds of pneumonia, leaving people with lung damage).

When she reported that the oxygen had dropped to 90 percent, I knew that the inflammatory process was worse in her lungs, causing damage and further causing shortness of breath, wheezing, and difficult breathing. I strongly advised her to go to the emergency room for further evaluation and intervention. Her symptoms were consistent with viral pneumonia from COVID-19. She did not want to go to the hospital. She had little kids at home. She had heard from the news that people went to the hospital with aggravated symptoms and ended up on a ventilator, and some people did not recover. In fact, just a few weeks before in our community, one friend in her mid-fifties had gone to the hospital and was told that she had waited "too long" and passed away in the hospital. People do not know how to assess themselves to go to the ER at the exact right time. Nobody knows. But I was able to treat symptoms and diseases more aggressively at home and prevented hospitalization, even in cases with severe symptoms.

Those who did seek help earlier, as soon as their symptoms started, received treatment per the algorithm created by Dr. Peter McCullough presented earlier for COVID-19, based on their clinical presentation and their report of having tested positive for COVID-19. Each patient was followed up closely by phone daily, or even twice a day, and according to their reports their condition improved day by day. They reported that in two to four days their fever went down, their oxygen levels went up, they coughed less, their muscle pain and headaches improved, and they started to get up and move around for the activities of daily living when they started treatment early—the first week of symptoms and viral disease.

CHAPTER 10

Covid-19 Patients' Restoration Testimonies

"For if you remain completely silent at this time, relief and deliverance will arise for the Jews from another place, but you and your father's house will perish. Yet who knows whether you have come to the kingdom for such a time as this?" (Esther 4:14-16 NKJV).

Recovery with Early Interventions

All this time during the pandemic, when the outbreak in our community started, I was terrified at the thought that I could not keep silent anymore. In my mind, the "war" started asking my conscious mind, "Whose voice do you follow? The voice of intimidation, or the voice of those desperate for help?" Immediately I recognized the voice of intimidation—the voice from the communist regime where I had to fight more than four decades ago: "You are about to lose your job if the communists find out that you are a person of faith in Christ Jesus, that you believe in the Word of God, that you go to church, that you go to prayer groups or Bible study..." I had to make the right decision now, as I did four decades ago in the communist country where I lived before I arrived in the USA: to obey the voice of the LORD. But in that "mind war," I focused on what I knew: that all of the medications I prescribed were approved in humans and had been used for a long time and were safe, and now I could use them "off-label" to save lives. What a privilege.

The voice of the Spirit was stronger. That voice inside of me was persistent, stating, "If you remain completely silent at this time, relief and deliverance for the sick people and their diseases will come from other places, but you will be held accountable that you did not listen to their cry in their desperation and did not help them in such a time as this." After my early and at-home interventions, patients started to send text messages telling me how good they felt after they started the treatment and early interventions at home, breaking the "sicken-in-place" method. So, I asked them to write their testimonies, and I included just a few here in this book to bring encouragement to those who live in crippling fear of COVID-19 symptoms and the diseases caused by it. And some of them mentioned ex-

DR. RODICA MALOS, DNP

actly those words, as patient R stated: "Thank you, Dr. Rodica, for your huge care and love, and for agreeing to be an Esther for such a time like this! You will have a big reward in heaven! Blessings & prayers!"

1. IR's testimony:

Dear Provider,

My name is IR, daughter of LR, who recently has received amazing care. I would like to thank you most profoundly for your diligent and godly care of my mother, and for the hope of health that came through your clinic! A special thank you to Dr. Rodica Malos.

My mother L had starting showing signs of CO-VID-19 sometime in early September: cough, fatigue, diarrhea, loss of taste and smell, low grade fever (100.1-101). She managed okay for a week, but her condition deteriorated quickly, to the point where she was very weak and barely could get out of bed, breathing heavier, with loss of appetite. We did the best we could for our mother: encouraged hourly fluids, food, and rest. It helped, but not nearly enough; she could get up, but weakness was still there.

Knowing of Dr. Rodica Malos (Romanian), I reached out to her to have my mother talk with her in

Romanian, and based on that phone call evaluation she received additional treatment with azithromycin, prednisone, and hydroxychloroquine. Within a few days of this treatment, my mother's condition and symptoms improved beyond belief! If I recall correctly, within three days of this treatment and the inhaler she was able to make soup for herself and her family that lives with her, and even encourage us with her positive spirit.

Praise God! Her breathing became lighter; coughs subsided but were with phlegm; her fever dissipated drastically; by the end of the week, she had a normal temperature with no fever-reducing drugs. Her appetite improved so much that she craved certain salads she made with fresh veggies from her garden. How wonderful is this! What joy came over our family, and we felt the spirit of stress and uncertainty flee from our home when Mom came out of the dark hour!

I know that in these challenging times, certain treatments these days are undermined if not restricted; I hope and pray that through this letter of encouragement and gratitude you will remain steadfast on the path of good health and support of those suffering.

With warmth and gratefulness on the behalf of LR, IR

2. V and R's testimony:

Dear Dr. Rodica Malos,

We can't find the words to express our thankfulness to God, Dr. Malos. The HCQ treatment worked right away! Even though my husband has problems with his heart; it is unbelievable!

No side effects, just healing and comfort right away! Even after the first tablet we felt the difference! To God be the glory! We are both well! We can enjoy our grandchildren!

And live a normal, blessed life! And this is just because we have brave enough doctors who really care about people, no matter how much pressure they have! May God bless Dr. Rodica Malos, who is a wonderful, kind, and very caring person.

Please keep doing what you are doing! You save lots of lives! Thank you!

3. A's testimony:

Hello, this is A, and through this testimony I want to encourage others that were affected by CO-VID-19 that there is hope! On the week of August 23-29, I had symptoms of fever on and off; I thought I had a cold, but after that week on September 1 I felt very weak, and I called to have an appointment with doctor Rodica Malos. After the appointment she prescribed me medication, and she prayed for me. After the second day of the treatment that I got, I had no more fever and my strength started to come back; the oxygen came back to normal, and in like five days I completed the treatment and I was fully recovered! Personally, I'm very thankful to God for your clinic and for Doctor Rodica Malos! Keep up the good work!

4. D and A's testimony:

We want to thank you from the bottom of our heart for treating both my husband and me during what possibly was the worst experience, faced with COVID-19. Both of us had more severe symptoms of COVID-19, and our symptoms were only worsening. We were at the point where we could hardly sit up for even a couple of minutes—we had the worst body aches of our life, fever, and headache. We were isolated, treating our symptoms with OTC and drinking lots of liquids to stay hydrated, but with everything we were doing we had reached a place where from one hour to the next my husband reached a point where he was hardly responding. That same day we had an appointment with Dr. Malos, and she prescribed hydroxychloroquine, zinc and Z-pack. Within two to three days we felt much better, and we were back on our feet. The way we had felt, I did not believe that, but Dr. Malos was right and truly a lifesaving mediator for us in fighting COVID-19. After a couple of days of taking hydroxychloroquine along with zinc and the Z-pack, we felt 90 percent better. We believe God sent Dr. Malos to provide us an escape from COVID-19 at the right time. May you continue to care, bless, and save people's lives with this treatment that saved our life.

God bless you,
D and A

5. S's testimony:

I am writing as a nurse and professor of nursing and a current caretaker for my parents, who within the last month had experienced signs and symptoms of COVID-19. My mother tested positive for COVID-19. They were assessed and treated by Dr. Rodica Malos immediately. Once the symptoms worsened, the treatment with hydroxychloroquine was started. Within twenty-four hours of being on the Zithromax and hydroxychloroquine regimen, both of my parents started feeling much better. The fever broke, their cough got better, and they started to improve.

I am certain that without this intervention, my parents would have needed to be hospitalized. In addition to those two medications, they took vitamin D, vitamin C, and zinc, all of which were recommendations made by Dr. Rodica Malos.

This treatment was imperative in the recovery of my parents, who are elderly: sixty-five and seventy years old. As a nurse and medical professional, I stand behind my testimony that this regimen was what saved my parents' lives and also kept them from going into the hospital. Please allow this treatment to continue to be prescribed for so many who are in need.

6. Pastor C's testimony:

Dear Doctor Rodica Malos,

I wanted to take the time to express my appreciation for the help that you have given me and my wife, as well as to several other members from our community.

As you know, on August 27 I contacted my doctor at KP, because I was not feeling well. Immediately, I was scheduled for a COVID-19 test and the result was positive.

Very concerned at the news, because of my history of sudden cardiac arrest, I contacted my doctor's office for treatment and advice. They basically told me to isolate and to wait for my symptoms to aggravate, and only then to call my doctor. In the meantime, I was told to drink tea with honey and to take Tylenol or other over-the-counter cold medications.

I could not believe what I was hearing! After all the warnings and all the stories from OHA about people dying from this virus, I considered that advice very inadequate.

For that reason, I called Dr. Malos for a second opinion. I was very fortunate to be able to speak to you on that same day and to receive treatment immediately, which included azithromycin, hydroxychloroquine, benzonatate, and zinc. After two days of taking this treatment my fever was gone, and in two more days, all my other symptoms had disappeared with the exception of some headaches and a sore throat. In less than a week, my energy level was back, and I was healed. After fourteen days of isolation, I returned safely to the community and to my work.

I want to thank you for being there for me and for all of your patients. I thank God for health professionals who care like you do.

Pastor C

During the outbreak of COVID-19 in our community, with the early interventions and patients recovering from mild and moderate symptoms, I heard powerful testimonies from each patient reporting their appreciation for the early treatment and their full recovery—thanking God for His goodness in their lives. I could distinguish the calm in the tone of their voice and the comfort received through early intervention.

Up to this day I receive testimonies from every patient whom I treated at home and who are so thankful and grateful to God that they found someone who cares, where they were able to receive care with the love of Christ in such as time as this.

Delayed Interventions Led to Hospitalizations

Below is an example of patients waiting too long at home with COVID-19 symptoms that got worse as a result of the "sicken-in-place" approach. When the symptoms got worse and they had difficulty breathing, in desperation they were seeking help at our primary care clinic on Friday evening when the clinic was closed. Patients who had waited too long needed to go to the ER, but damage was done to their lungs already from the inflammation process of the cytokine storm as a result of the immune system's response to the multiplication of the virus in the second phase of the disease. They needed to be hospitalized for more aggressive and stronger treatment, because they did develop viral pneumonia and further complications. They needed a longer time to recover. Their health condition and quality of life are not the same after their lungs were damaged from the debris and residuals from the inflammatory process in the alveoli that caused pneumonia.

Patients who developed pneumonia from COVID-19 infection broke my heart, knowing that they were the victims of the "sicken-in-place" approach that led to increased severity of the symptoms and fast deterioration, leading to lung damage and pneumonia, becoming hospital-dependent as a result. If they had early access to HCQ, antibiotics, steroids, bronchodilators, inhalers, and oxygen supplementation as recommended in the algorithm presented earlier, they could have avoided hospitalization and further damage to their body, soul, and spirit. Their health conditions and quality of life would be different.

Looking back on my experience in a short period of time with more than a hundred patients treated at home early, when symptoms started, and who recovered completely, I am confident that by providing early interventions, we could reduce hundreds of thousands of hospitalizations and prevent hundreds of thousands of deaths in the United States of America as well as in many countries around the world and avoid so many losses economically, financially, emotionally, intellectually, mentally, and spiritually.

CHAPTER 11

God Speaks in Medicine

"Your ears shall hear a word behind you, saying, 'This is the way, walk in it,' whenever you turn to the right hand or whenever you turn to the left" (Isaiah 30:21 NKJV).

Amazing Way of God's Work

After hearing so many testimonies from patients who recovered from COVID-19 through early interventions, I reflected back on God's amazing way of working to connect me with a small clinic (that will remain anonymous for confidentiality reasons). He guided me with His small voice to the right place to practice during the pandemic, to save lives. It happened that my husband and I took a sabbatical year after working for about twenty-eight years in our very demanding business, which physically and emotionally drained our energy from 24/7 relentless work, providing care to people with multiple chronic conditions and challenging behaviors. When we returned from our time of rest, I found out that Portland Adventist Community Service Health Clinic (PACS-HC), where I had been volunteering for about sixteen years as a general practitioner in primary care, had changed its profile and transitioned to a dental and ophthalmological clinic.

As a result, I started to pray for God to give me guidance and to direct my steps to a new clinic, where I could continue to volunteer my time helping the most vulnerable and needy people. After a few months in the process of seeking God's leading, through the power of the Holy Spirit I heard an instant, fulgurating voice in my head say, "Dr. S." I was pleasantly surprised, because I had met Dr. S more than ten years ago, when we wanted to learn a new program from his practice to adapt to PACS clinic. I remembered that he prayed when we had a problem with the program on his computer, and the computer worked right away. That kind of bold prayer had an impact on my prayer life and I did remember him vividly for that prayer, even after ten years. I knew he was a man of faith and prayer.

I Listened to the Small Voice

I paid attention to the "small voice" that resonated in my head because I knew God was speaking to me. I'd had that experience before, and I had to listen and obey. Prophet Isaiah assures us, "Your ears shall hear a word behind you, saying, 'This is the way, walk in it,' whenever you turn to the right hand or whenever you turn to the left" (Isaiah 30:21 NKJV).

I contacted Dr. S's clinic right away and connected with the staff for application and orientation. A few weeks after proceeding with the paperwork and job orientation, the news about COVID-19 shocked everybody. After a few weeks of working with patients, the clinic closed, and telehealth was implemented. I was very happy that I could provide medical care for patients even via telemedicine to be able to help, as much as I could, people in need of medical care. God's divine intervention to connect me with Dr. S's clinic had been orchestrated ahead of time, so I could act and follow His guidance to help hundreds of people in terrible distress in the pandemic time. Only God knew what was coming over the earth, and in our city and community. He prepared me ahead of time just for that. God knows the end from the beginning. I am glad that I listened to the "small voice."

PART II

CHAPTER 12

Science and Beyond

Where Is the Evidence?

"For the LORD gives wisdom; from His mouth come knowledge and understanding" (Proverbs 2:6 NKJV).

Being led by the Spirit during the pandemic time does not mean that I underestimated science or lowered the standards of care. Our practice in medicine is guided by science. Our life is surrounded by science. God created science. But science is not God. God is above science. He gives wisdom to people on earth to develop science. He is sovereign and has the highest authority, and He wants us to look beyond science when we are in crises—especially in a pandemic time, when we do not have time to wait for the best evidence from randomized clinical trials. In those extreme situations we depend on God, our Creator. We read in Proverbs

2:6, "For the LORD gives wisdom; from His mouth come knowledge and understanding" (Proverbs 2:6 NKJV).

Dr.Vinay Prasad, MD, MPH, a practicing hematologist-oncologist and Associate Professor of Medicine in the Division of Epidemiology and Biostatistics at the University of California, San Francisco, stated on MedPage Today: "I love being a scientist and researcher, but I must admit that scientists have no special ability to adjudicate value judgements, and as such, we can never follow the science; the hard decisions are up to all of us. Just out: I offer eight theses about science:

1. Science is not policy
2. Credentialism is not science
3. Science needs testable hypotheses
4. Science is not censoring
5. Science is not a popularity contest
6. Science applies criticism fairly
7. Observational studies are often unreliable
8. Pragmatism is needed"[19]

In primary care health clinics, primary care providers are disengaged in caring for patients with COVID-19, sending them home to wait until the symptoms from the COVID-19 infection get worse and to then go to the ER and hospital for further evaluation and treatment. I did feel chills on my spine again from threats from the authorities that we must wait for randomized clinical trials to develop the best evidence that could not be developed in such a short time, when the novel virus COVID-19 spread so fast and killed hundreds of thousands of people. I agree 100 percent with the authorities that we should obey science—by title, I am a scientist and I love science—but in such a short period of time during a pandemic, there is no time to develop science to guide our practices for anything we do to prevent the spread of the virus and to prevent death from the diseases caused by the virus. People are dying while we are waiting for clinical trials that can take years to be accomplished.

Using Alternative Approaches While Waiting

The reality is that the cruelty of the virus is felt by everyone, and it is killing people in front of our eyes, and we have no time to wait for randomized controlled trials that take a long time for a quality study and are impractical in such short period of time. Alternative approaches are extremely important to save people's lives during a pandemic. We are left with common sense, and with the knowledge and experience of past qualitative studies and scientific evidence, and positive outcomes from our experience in our practice that the authorities denied. I relived my experience from a communist country, where I lived under the oppression of a communist regime for more than three decades, by experiencing flashbacks from communist propaganda that we were not allowed to engage in saving souls by telling them that the wages of sin is death. At that time, under the communist regime, I was told that if I talked to people about my hope in Jesus Christ I would lose my job and I would be left with no resources and sentenced to death. No social support services were provided during communism. If you lose your job, you die from hunger by starving to death.

Now again during the pandemic, I had to live in the dark of terror, with no solutions for our sick patients—abandoning them when they needed us the most due to a lack of randomized clinical trials during the pandemic. I felt the condemnation from other practitioners in primary care who were denying treatment to patients with COVID-19, telling them to take OTC preparations, use home remedies, and drink fluids. That was the minimum you could do using common sense if mild symptoms started. We do not have science for those kinds of approaches either. The media continued to suppress information that encouraged providers and patients about early interventions to save lives. For example, listening to the media and reading articles with so much negativism about President Trump's assertion about hydroxychloroquine, I had to find more evidence about this medication. Searching for more evidence, I found that "in 2005, the CDC Special Pathogens Branch described three mechanisms by which chloroquine might work and have both a prophylactic and therapeutic role in coronavirus infections. More than 20 relevant studies have been published in journals indexed in PubMed between Jan 28 and April 20, 2020."[20]

The top doctors were even looking at studies done in different countries to learn from other experts and scientists around the world, to obtain the best data to implement in our practice to decrease death rates, as is described in the following findings: "Additionally, AAPS is compiling observational results reported from China, France, South Korea, Algeria, and the U.S. Of 2,333 patients treated with HCQ, 2,137 or 91.6 percent improved clinically. There were 63 deaths, all but 11 in a single retrospective report from the Veterans Administration where the patients were severely ill. Apr 27 data shows that U.S. COVID-19 death rates are at least eight times higher than in countries with early and prophylactic use of HCQ."[21]

More and more studies are showing good results when HCQ is used early. "The website c19study.com summarizes more than 130 studies of HCQ, which are overwhelmingly positive particularly when HCQ is used early, as well as studies of other drugs and vitamin D."[22]

Extensive Evidence

Dr. Harvey Risch reported that seven clinical studies showed significant benefits from HCQ around the world and in the USA. "There is extensive evidence that HCQ, when used within the first five days of symptom onset, produces a sharp and statistically significant reduction in hospitalization and mortality. Seven controlled, well-conducted clinical studies show this: 636 outpatients in São Paulo, Brazil; 199 clinic patients in Marseille, France; 717 patients across a large HMO network in Brazil; 226 nursing-home patients in Marseille; 1,247 outpatients in New Jersey; 100 long-term care institution patients in Andorra (between France and Spain); and 7,892 patients across Saudi Arabia. All of these studies pertain to the early treatment of high-risk outpatients, and all showed 50% or higher reductions in hospitalization or death. Not a single fatal cardiac arrhythmia attributable to the HCQ was reported among these thousands of patients. In addition, a new summary analysis of five randomized controlled trials has also shown a statistically significant outpatient benefit, proving the case."[23]

Dr. Vladimir Zelenko, who is saving thousands of lives with early interventions in his practice, demonstrated that "the well-tolerated 5-day triple therapy resulted in a significantly lower hospitalization rate and less fatalities with no reported cardiac side effects compared with relevant public reference data of untreated patients. The magnitude of the results can substantially elevate the relevance of early use, low dose hydroxy-chloroquine, especially in combination with zinc. This data can be used to inform ongoing pandemic response policies as well as future clinical trials."[24]

And demonstrated, "For outpatients with a median of only 4 days after onset of symptoms, COVID-19 represents a totally different disease and needs to be managed and treated differently. A simple to perform outpatient risk stratification, as shown here, allows rapid treatment decisions and treatment with the triple therapy of zinc, low dose HCQ, and azithromycin and may prevent a large number of hospitalizations and probably deaths during the SARS-CoV-2 pandemic. This might also help to avoid overwhelming of the health care systems."[25]

Dr. Zelenko's Protocol for Early Intervention

Below is Dr. Vladimir Zelenko's protocol presented on Twitter:

@zev_dr, "The Zelenko Protocol Treatment Plan for Patients with COVID-19 symptoms: Prehospital Management."

Fundamental Principles

Treat patients based on clinical suspicion as soon as possible, preferably within the first 5 days of symptoms. Perform PCR testing, but do not withhold treatment pending results.

Risk Stratify Patients

Low risk patient - Younger than 60, no comorbidities, and clinically stable

High risk patient - Older than 60, younger than 60 with comorbidities, or clinically unstable

Treatment Options

Low risk patients - over the counter options:

1. Elemental Zinc 50mg 1 time a day for 7 days
2. Quercetin 500mg 2 times a day for 7 days **or** Epigallocatechin-gallate (EGCG) 400mg 1 time a day for 7 days
3. Vitamin C 1000mg 1 time a day for 7 days
4. Rest, oral fluids and close follow-up with doctor

High risk patients

1. Elemental Zinc 50mg 1 time a day for 7 days
2. Hydroxychloroquine (HCQ) 200mg 2 times a day for 7 days. If HCQ not available, Quercetin 500mg 3 times a day for 7 days **or** EGCG 400mg 2 times a day for 7 days

3. Azithromycin 500mg 1 time a day for 5 days **or** Doxycycline 100mg 2 times a day for 7 days
4. Vitamin C 1000mg 1 time a day for 7 days
5. Rest, oral fluids and close follow-up with doctor

Additional treatment options. Should be uniquely custom tailored for every patient.

1. Ivermectin 6mg 2 times a day for 1 day
2. Budesonide 1mg/2cc solution via nebulizer 2 times a day for 7 days
3. Dexamethasone 6mg 1 time a day for 7 days
4. Blood thinners (i.e. Lovenox)
5. Home oxygen
6. Home IV fluids

IF POSSIBLE, KEEP PATIENTS OUT OF THE HOSPITAL[26]

Mary Beth Pfeiffer, in "This Doctor has COVID-19. He Has a Plan. For All of Us" on Oct 30, 2020, stated that Dr. McCullough, who had treated more than a hundred COVID-19 patients, had his own experience with the viral infection. He said, "You may have noticed that I sneezed a little bit through the presentation. Yesterday I got the bad news that I myself have developed COVID-19."

He went from physician to patient, in an early treatment protocol that he helped design. The protocol is a collaboration of about two dozen U.S. and Italian researchers; it was published in August in the *American Journal of Medicine* and since updated. Like other protocols—originating in France, California, and New York—the regimen firmly rejects the current "sicken-in-place" approach that leaves COVID-19 patients untreated until, intensely ill, they land in a hospital.

Dr. McCullough's Personal Treatment Regimen, as of Day 7

- Ivermectin, 12 mg a day for 3 days
- Hydroxychloroquine, 200 mg twice a day for 5-30 days in an open label safety study
- Zinc sulfate, 220 mg a day all days
- Vitamin C, 3000 mg a day all days
- Vitamin D3, 5,000 IU all days
- Azithromycin, 250 mg twice a day all days
- Aspirin, 325 mg a day all days
- Colchicine or placebo, as part of the COLCORONA research study medication for 30 days
- Prednisone, 60 mg five days (holding it for backup if pulmonary symptoms worsen)
- Apixaban, 5 mg twice a day (holding it for backup if pulmonary symptoms worsen)[27]

Ivermectin was mentioned in the above protocols by both Dr. Zelenko and Dr. McCullough and used for early intervention. The FLCCC Alliance also discovered that ivermectin has anti-viral and anti-inflammatory properties, improving patients' symptoms from the COVID-19 virus. "The FLCCC then recently discovered that ivermectin, an anti-parasitic medicine, has highly potent anti-viral and anti-inflammatory properties against COVID-19. They then identified repeated, consistent, large magnitude improvements in clinical outcomes in multiple, large, randomized and observational controlled trials in both prophylaxis and treatment of COVID-19."[28]

Pierre Kory, MD et. al. discovered that it "resulted from multiple, large 'natural experiments' that occurred when various city mayors and regional health ministries within South American countries initiated 'ivermectin distribution' campaigns to their citizen populations in the hopes the drug would prove effective. The tight, reproducible, temporally associated decreases in case counts and case fatality rates in each of those regions, compared to nearby regions without such campaigns, suggest that ivermectin may prove to be a global solution to the pandemic. This was further evidenced by the recent incorporation of ivermectin as a prophylaxis and treatment agent for COVID-19 in the national treatment guidelines of Belize, Macedonia, and the state of Uttar Pradesh in Northern India, populated by 210 million people."[29]

Dr. Pierre Kory's experience in tirelessly providing care to patients with COVID-19 in the ICU—and seeing many of the patients dying under his care due to complications from COVID-19 symptoms—led him to the hard work of searching for data from different parts of the world to access information about the effectiveness of ivermectin, which could be a solution to stop the pandemic. I heard one of his interviews where he was emotionally drained, almost crying, begging the Senate to review the data that he had obtained to prove that ivermectin is an effective drug for COVID-19 symptoms, providing benefits to treat the disease and for prophylactic treatment.

The last patient who experienced advanced symptoms from COVID-19 whose oxygen levels dropped below 88 percent at night was extremely tired and weak and in desperation for medical care. It was too late to start HCQ, but she followed the protocol mentioned above, and I added (to her current treatment) ivermectin 12 mg by mouth every day for 3 days per Peter A. Mc-Cullough, MD, MPH's protocol. The patient's oxygen levels increased from 88 percent to 93 percent after the first dose in less than twenty-four hours, to 95 percent after the second dose, and to 97 percent after the third dose. The patient recovered well and was happy and praised the Lord for His mighty intervention through medications that we have available and that are affordable. She was very happy, because she was scared to death at the thought that she needed to go to the ER and be hospitalized for severe symptoms from COVID-19. This is another example of great benefits from the protocols and algorithms developed by top doctors with lifetime experience, using medications to treat symptoms based on the pathophysiology of the diseases caused by COVID-19. My heart is full of thanks to God and those prominent physicians, general practitioners, and specialists who advocate for the most vulnerable population suffering from COVID-19.

CHAPTER 13

Medical Justice

A Way Prepared

"No temptation has overtaken you except such as is common to man; but God is faithful, who will not allow you to be tempted beyond what you are able, but with the temptation will also make the way of escape, that you may be able to bear it" (1 Corinthians 10:13 NKJV).

In the darkest time during this pandemic, God prepared the way for early interventions so patients could escape the trials from the virus. The trial came unexpectedly, but God inspired doctors with expertise and experience in medicine to discover the solutions for the symptoms from the virus for patients to be treated with early interventions and treatment. God inspired many doctors to develop protocols to be followed even for prophylactic prevention of the diseases from the virus.

I believe that to stop the early interventions at home available for patients in primary care and to use the "sicken-in-place" approach is a medical injustice for patients who are suffering with severe symptoms at home until they become so sick they are fainting, very weak, unable to get out of bed to perform the activities of daily living, dependent, trying to survive at home, terrified that if they go to the hospital they will not come back home, as many patients said when they expressed their frustration when treatment at home had been refused, and they verbalized their fear that tormented them.

Withholding Early Intervention is Dangerous

While I was meditating on what happens during this time of pandemic when we withhold early treatments and interventions at home from people who are in great distress due to sickness, crying out to God—and some die in the hospital as a result—the scripture came to my mind of Abel and Cain's story from ancient times, written in God's Word as follows: "So the LORD said to Cain, 'Why are you angry? And why has your countenance fallen? If you do well, will you not be accepted? And if you do not do well, sin lies at the door. And its desire is for you, but you should rule over it.' Now Cain talked with Abel his brother; and it came to pass, when they were in the field, that Cain rose up against Abel his brother and killed him. Then the LORD said to Cain, 'Where is Abel your brother?' He said, 'I do not know. Am I my brother's keeper?' And He said, 'What have you done? The voice of your brother's blood cries out to Me from the ground. So now you are cursed from the earth, which has opened its mouth to receive your brother's blood from your hand. When you till the ground, it shall no longer yield its strength to you. A fugitive and a vagabond you shall be on the earth'" (Genesis 4:6-12 NKJV). In the health care field, we all have responsibilities to do well for our patients and to treat their symptoms from COVID-19 and their diseases when they are in physical and psychological distress, in order to be accepted as God's servants, doing what we were trained for.

Patient's Life Does Matter

In my opinion, we must think in terms that each patient's life matters. Recently, I received a call from a Romanian Christian lady who was in desperation for her husband's life—a healthy, strong man who was infected with COVID-19. In the first week of mild and moderate symptoms he got no early intervention treatment from the primary care provider, and his symptoms got worse as time passed, and his oxygen levels dropped to 90-92 percent (from 96-99 percent, the normal range). He went to the ER and was admitted to the hospital, and in five days he was placed on a ventilator, and he died two weeks later and left behind a devastated family. That is an example of a very active, healthy sixty-year-old male whose life could have been saved with early interventions. I did cry and grieve with that dear family. I was thinking, *Who are we in primary care to withhold early interventions from sick patients when they need us the most?*

We tell them to wait at home until they are sick enough to go to the emergency room. By that time, damage to the vital organs has already been done by the inflammation process and the micro thrombosis caused by such an aggressive virus that multiplies in the first week and then provokes the immune system to overreact and to release the cytokine storm, causing inflammation and blood clots, and the chance to survive is diminished. Even if the patients survive, they are left with post COVID-19 symptoms from the inflammatory phase and residuals from debris from the disease process of the virus. We must provide care to every single patient with symptoms from COVID-19 with that truth in our mind—that every single patient's life matters.

Prevent Covid-19 Measures

Do Not Sorrow; Take Action

"Then he said to them, 'Go your way, eat the fat, drink the sweet, and send portions to those for whom nothing is prepared; for this day is holy to our Lord. Do not sorrow, for the joy of the LORD is your strength'" (Nehemiah 8:10 NKJV).

Prevention is the key in every disease that affects humans. During COVID-19, it is important to use common sense and to follow instructions for preventative measures such as wearing a mask where social distancing is not possible, social distancing if people are sick, washing hands frequently, disinfecting, avoiding big crowds, avoiding sick people, staying home if you are sick, and improving your immune system. These are all good practices to prevent contracting the virus. However, the uncertainty of how long all those practices will be prolonged affects our society directly and indirectly, leading to anxiety and depression with long-term consequences.

By wearing masks, people miss seeing others' smiles. Our mirror neurons in our brain have the role of helping us to smile when others are smiling at us. In Romans chapter 12, verse 15, we read, "Rejoice with those who rejoice, and weep with those who weep" (Romans 12:15 NKJV). Joy is one of the most powerful emotions that brings healing to our body, spirit, and soul. Joy is the antidote for sadness and depression. The reward mechanism in our brain is activated when we are full of joy and dopamine is released, improving our motivation for the activities of daily living and everyday life. Serotonin and endorphins, oxytocin, and other neurochemicals are released in the body to restore our health and to keep us healthy. Smiling is extremely important in our daily life, to prevent the anxiety and depression that affect our body, soul, and spirit in a negative way. Joy brings health and strength to our being. The Bible teaches us about the importance of being happy and rejoicing always. A great example is written in Nehemiah about the joy of the Lord that is our strength in times of sorrow and distress. "Then he said to them, 'Go your way, eat the fat, drink the sweet, and send portions to those for whom nothing is prepared; for this day is holy to our Lord. Do not sorrow, for the joy of the LORD is your strength'" (Nehemiah 8:10 NKJV).

After almost one year of the pandemic situation worldwide, there are still many things to learn about the transmission of the virus COVID-19 and the severity caused by it. That is the dilemma for all experts and scientists, and all professional people working in the health care field. Due to a lack of specific, scientific evidence, people are more anxious and more concerned, not having clear solutions.

We must emphasize some aspects of the transmission of this virus; the signs and symptoms that develop after COVID-19 exposure and infection; the signs and symptoms of an emergency; how to protect ourselves to prevent infection with COVID-19; the importance of our immune system in fighting this unpredictable virus; and co-morbidities prevention and the complications caused by COVID-19 in persons with those co-morbidities.

Using the Spirit of Wisdom

"He who gets wisdom loves his own soul; he who keeps understanding will find good" (Proverbs 19:8 NKJV).

Throughout this pandemic, people have endless questions due to the unknowns and uncertainties they face. We can have peace that passes all understanding when we get wisdom from above during this hard time through the pandemic. Here are short responses to the most common questions people have about virus CO-VID-19 and the diseases caused by it. The CDC displays all of these recommendation on the internet, easily accessible to any person.

1. What do we need to know about COVID-19?
   a. How is it transmitted?
   We learned from the CDC that:
   - The COVID-19 virus is transmitted from person to person at a distance of less than six feet.
   - It is transmitted through respiratory particles produced by an infected person when they are coughing, sneezing, or talking.
   - These particles get into our mouth and nose and are inhaled into our lungs from the particles spread by infected persons in the atmosphere around us.
   - Some persons can spread the virus if they do not have symptoms.

   b. How fast is this virus transmitted?
   -COVID-19 is transmitted faster and more easily than influenza, and more slowly than measles, which is very contagious.

Signs and Symptoms

c. What are the signs and symptoms?
- Fever
- Dry cough (sometimes can be productive)
- Sore throat
- Shortness of breath (many patients will report, "I cannot breathe"; others state, "I cannot get enough air in my lungs," or "The air is staying at the entrance of my lungs," or "I have pressure in my chest" or "There is burning inside my chest when I breathe" or "burning inside of the upper back," etc.)
- Hypoxia (when the oxygen level drops from 97 to 89), in many cases seven to eight days into the progression of the disease. Those people need to be on alert to go to the hospital right away, because the oxygenation is compromised in vital organs, tissues, and cells, and this creates multi-organ failure and death. People may try to use a nebulizer and an oxygen machine at home. But even with those interventions, if the oxygen level drops below 90 percent, people must go to the hospital for further evaluation and interventions.
- Chest pain
- Chest pressure
- Cyanosis, bluish lips, skin discoloration

- Chills and sweats
- Headache
- Pink eye
- Muscle and joint pain (many patients report that "it is like someone is pulling my flesh away from me") causing excruciating pain
- Syncope (people get up to perform the activities of daily living and fall on the floor, fainting)
- Extreme fatigue and tiredness, unable to get up to use the bathroom
- Dizziness
- Anorexia
- Smell and taste loss
- Nausea, vomiting
- Diarrhea

All of those symptoms are real. The majority of those symptoms were experienced by the patients who sought interventions and treatment. Because COVID-19 symptoms manifest in these many ways, every person's condition is different, presenting at a mild, moderate, and severe level.

"A new study by researchers at the University College London revealed that 86 percent of people who tested positive for COVID-19 did not have virus symptoms, such as cough, fever, and loss of taste or smell."[30]

Our body is created in a very complex way to fight trillions of viruses' cells and stay strong, not even exhibiting any symptoms at all. The psalmist wrote about God's complex work in our body 3,500 years ago, stating, "Thank you for making me so wonderfully complex! Your workmanship is marvelous—how well I know it" (Psalm 139:14 NLT).

CHAPTER 15

Signs and Symptoms of an Emergency

When to Seek Emergency Medical Attention

Mr. J, during his experience with COVID-19, was in great distress; while staying at home waiting for the symptoms to get worse, he called me and asked how he would know when to call 911 or when to go to the emergency room. He was consumed with worries, not knowing when was the right time to seek medical attention. Many patients are in terrible distress because they do not know when to go to the hospital, because many patients go to the ER and are sent home because they are not sick enough to be hospitalized. That creates confusion and psychological distress.

This is what the CDC recommends for an emergency situation:

Look for **emergency warning signs*** of COVID-19. If someone is showing any of these signs, **seek emergency medical care immediately:**
- Trouble breathing
- Persistent pain or pressure in the chest
- New confusion
- Inability to wake or stay awake
- Bluish lips or face

*This list is not all possible symptoms. Please call your medical provider for any other symptoms that are severe or concerning to you. Call 911 or call ahead to your local emergency facility: Notify the operator that you are seeking care for someone who has or may have COVID-19.[31]

Many patients develop difficulty breathing after their lungs are affected by COVID-19, but they do not realize that. When I interviewed patients for their symptoms when they called me to report that they had tested positive, I asked if they had a cough. Their response many times was no, then after a few more questions I would hear them coughing between words on the phone. They were not even aware that they did have a dry cough. Others had a "wet sound" and a "tired larynx" when they talked that indicated that they had symptoms but were not aware of them.

I strongly advised patients to check and monitor their oxygen levels every day, even two to three times a day, using a pulse oximeter (a very small device that can be found at a pharmacy or medical supply store, or even ordered on Amazon online). When oxygen levels drop below 96 percent, it is an indication that the virus has multiplied, provoking the immune system to cause an inflammatory process in the lungs. The damage in the lungs starts from the bottom, at the alveolar level where the exchange of oxygen and carbon dioxide happens, and the oxygenation is impaired by the damaged alveoli by the virus' multiplication in the lung cells. That is the time to be hypervigilant and to watch for more decline in oxygen levels, and signs of hypoxia such as cyanosis and bluish lips and face, and to call the family doctor or go directly to the ER.

The majority of patients with compulsive cough episodes, dyspnea, and oxygen levels decreasing to 89 percent can be treated with steroids such as prednisone or dexamethasone, inhalers, nebulizers, and oxygen supplementation in their own home if they have no life-threatening conditions. If the patient's condition declines to where they are unable to get up to use the bathroom, develop severe chest pain, or have increased fever of more than 101 degrees Fahrenheit even with maximum treatment of Tylenol or NSAIDs (nonsteroidal anti-inflammatory drugs) such as ibuprofen or Advil and others, they need to go to the hospital.

Some patients experienced syncope: one patient reported that she went to the bathroom and fainted when used the toilet; another patient went to shave and fainted in the bathroom, etc. One patient's blood pressure dropped to 78/46 and he got very weak, so that he could not stand up. He was found by his wife on the floor in the morning. Other patients reported that they were so sick that they were unable to stand up and move around to perform the activities of daily living, or to cook for themselves. When I asked them to go to the emergency room, they refused. Some patients expressed concern that if they went to the hospital their condition would deteriorate more, and they would end up on a ventilator and die. In those situations, I had to step in and start treatment right away, and their lives were saved by God's grace only.

Call Your Doctor and Go to the Emergency Room Right Away

"But the wisdom that is from above is first pure, then peaceable, gentle, willing to yield, full of mercy and good fruits, without partiality and without hypocrisy" (James 3:17 NKJV).

If you experience trouble breathing, persistent pain or pressure in the chest, new confusion, inability to wake or stay awake, bluish lips or face, even if you have received any kind of treatment for early intervention or if you take a prophylactic treatment, you must go to the hospital (ER). People must know that each case is different—because each person is uniquely created, with unique DNA with instructions for life, and a unique immune system response when activated by the virus. Each person's genetic makeup is different and responds differently to the COVID-19 virus infection.

Dr. Blaylock stated, "This is somewhat of an unusual virus in that for the vast majority of people infected by the virus, one experiences either no illness (asymptomatic) or very little sickness."[32] But many patients can become very sick, with life-threatening symptoms.

Signs and symptoms can manifest two to fourteen days after exposure to the virus and then will follow its course, according to your health condition and your immunity to fight the virus back.

Pay attention to the signs and symptoms of COVID-19.

I give patients the following instructions, but more instructions can be added as appropriate:

1. Patient instructed to follow CDC recommendations for isolation to prevent spreading of the virus.

2. Patient instructed to go to ER if:
    * temperature is over 101 (even if taking OTC meds for fever)
    * if respiration rate is more than 30 breaths per minute (even if taking bronchodilators via inhalers or nebulizers)
    * oxygen level is lower than 90%, (even with oxygen supplementation)
    * if cyanotic
    * if experiencing chest pain, chest pressure, shortness of breath, increased fatigue, increased dizziness, syncope, fainting, and other unusually severe symptoms.
    * Hold medication if heart rate is lower than 60 beats/min or if experiencing irregular heartbeats, and contact medical provider immediately
    * Take aspirin 325 mg daily to prevent blood clots during COVID-19 symptoms

VERY IMPORTANT: Talk to your doctor about all your signs and symptoms during this pandemic period, and after the pandemic is over, to detect any residuals from the diseases caused by COVID-19. Do not ignore any symptoms, as they may give you signals about damage done in your body by the virus even after the pandemic is over.

There is nothing new under sun since creation: "What has been will be again, what has been done will be done again; there is nothing new under the sun" (Ecclesiastes 1:9 NIV). God is even in the middle of a pandemic to give us directions for early interventions and how to protect ourselves from the COVID-19 virus.

How to Protect Yourself and Others

Isolation in the Bible:

"Go, my people, enter your rooms and shut the doors behind you; hide yourselves for a little while until his wrath has passed by. See, the Lord is coming out of his dwelling to punish the people of the earth for their sins. The earth will disclose the blood shed on it; the earth will conceal its slain no longer" (Isaiah 26:20-21 NIV).

As we have all learned from CDC recommendations, the best way to prevent infection with COVID-19 is to avoid exposure to the virus by:

- Maintaining at least six feet of distance (the most important measure to prevent transmission of this virus).
- Washing your hands frequently with soap and water. If soap and water are not available, use sanitary solutions that contain at least 60 percent alcohol.

- Avoiding touching eyes, nose, and mouth with unwashed hands.
- Disinfecting very well the surfaces you touch frequently.

Avoid Close Contact

From ancient times we have learned that we must avoid people with contagious diseases and that they must be isolated, as God told Moses and Aaron in Leviticus 13: "The Lord said to Moses and Aaron, 'When anyone has a swelling or a rash or a shiny spot on their skin that may be a defiling skin disease, they must be brought to Aaron the priest or to one of his sons who is a priest. The priest is to examine the sore on the skin, and if the hair in the sore has turned white and the sore appears to be more than skin deep, it is a defiling skin disease. When the priest examines that person, he shall pronounce them ceremonially unclean. If the shiny spot on the skin is white but does not appear to be more than skin deep and the hair in it has not turned white, the priest is to isolate the affected person for seven days. On the seventh day the priest is to examine them, and if he sees that the sore is unchanged and has not spread in the skin, he is to isolate them for another seven days'" (Leviticus 13:1-5 NIV).

It is very interesting that our usual treatment regimen for early intervention for COVID-19 virus infections and symptoms is five to seven days, and if the patient continues to experience symptoms, we repeat the treatment for five to seven more days. That portion of Scripture was written about 3,500 years ago.

How can you protect yourself?
- Avoid contact with sick persons.
- Keep a distance of at least six feet between persons from outside, but even members of your own family.
- You must keep in mind that even persons with no symptoms can transmit the virus.
- Avoid group gatherings during the outbreak of the virus.
- Respect distance with other people, and especially those at high risk to get sick, and especially people at high risk to develop complications: old people; persons with heart disease, lung conditions, diabetes; persons who are immunocompromised or on immunosuppressant medication; and others.
- Cover your face with a mask or scarf when you are around other people.
- You can spread COVID-19 to other people even when you are not sick.
- Every person must cover mouth, nose when going in public, shopping.

- It is contraindicated to use a mask for children under two years old, people with respiratory problems, and those unable to take off the mask without assistance.
- The mask has the role of protecting those around you if you are infected with COVID-19.
- The mask does not replace the distancing method.
- You do not need to wear your mask if you are alone in your private space.
- Always cover your mouth and nose when you cough or sneeze with a napkin, or cough or sneeze into your elbow.
- Throw into the garbage all tissues used to cover cough or sneezing.
- Immediately wash your hands with soap and water for twenty seconds.
- For disinfection, use solutions that contain at least 60 percent alcohol if soap and water are not available.
- Disinfect daily all the surfaces frequently used such as: tables, doorknobs, light switches, cooking surfaces, desks, telephones, keyboards.
- Disinfect daily toilets, handles, faucets, sinks.
- Clean dirty surfaces first with detergents or soap and water, then disinfect.
- Use household disinfectants from stores.

- Verify at all times all the recommendations from the National Centers for Disease Control and Prevention.[33]

Outdoor activities are recommended for health promotion and disease prevention. But during the pandemic, due to the airflow with respiratory droplets, being around those who walk and run even in outdoor activities can lead to viral infections. The CDC recommendations are that distancing is a great practice, but those who are walking must keep sixteen feet of distance and those who are running must keep thirty-two feet of distance, because the respiratory droplets in the pathways are denser in that narrow corridor of those who walk and run.[34]

CHAPTER 16

Strong Immune System—Fight Covid-19

"Now there are varieties of gifts, but the same Spirit; and there are varieties of service, but the same Lord; and there are varieties of activities, but it is the same God who empowers them all in everyone" (1 Corinthians 12:4-6 ESV).

Metabolic Syndrome (Hypertension, Diabetes, Dyslipidemia)

At this time there is no clear evidence nor pharmacological strategies to prevent and to treat 100 percent the disease caused by COVID-19, and nobody knows exactly the time when this alarming situation with this virus will end. The most important thing at this time is to explore strategies to improve our immune system to fight this unpredictable and "invisible enemy," and to take prophylactic treatment and vaccination when available and appropriate.

To prevent severe complications caused by COVID-19, it is extremely important to reduce obesity and metabolic syndrome (hypertension, diabetes, dyslipidemia). In my first book, Find Your Peace: Supernatural Solutions Beyond Science for Fear, Anxiety, and Depression, I wrote in detail about how to prevent metabolic syndrome through lifestyle changes and stress management of fear, anxiety, and depression. Checking blood pressure, blood sugar, and cholesterol levels is extremely important to managing and controlling them with a healthy diet, exercise, and medication as necessary

It is important to check vitamin levels and to address all vitamin deficiencies with fresh fruits and vegetables and probiotics. A healthy diet and hydration are extremely necessary. A balanced diet with a variety of healthy nutrients is extremely important. It is extremely important to seek medical advice about micronutrient supplementation and calorie intake with healthy nutrients for each person, according to their own condition.

Strengthen the Immune System

It is recommended:

- Using multiple vitamins plays a huge role in strengthening the immune system for vulnerable persons with vitamin deficiencies, such as persons with restrictions in their diet: vegetarians, infants, children, adolescents, pregnant women, breastfeeding women, and the elderly.

- Many people have deficiencies of micronutrients such as vitamin D due to lack of sun exposure. It is important to use vitamin D 2000 IU daily. But the level of vitamin D must be checked by the family doctor through labs.

I mentioned that Dr Crandall, in his book Fight Back, makes recommendations for supplements to optimize the immune system. He stated, "To fight back against COVID-19, you need every weapon you can lay your hands on, and this means taking supplements, which can give you an important nutritional edge. These recommendations can strengthen your immune system to help fight off COVID-19... These are the essential supplements you need to keep your immune system strong. They are also useful if you feel the symptoms of a cold, the flu, or even what you suspect might be COVID-19 coming on. It's also always important to take a multivitamin every day to cover any deficiencies you might have of which you are unaware."[35]

For a healthy immune system, take daily:
- Vitamin C 1,000 mg

- Vitamin D 5,000 IU (your vitamin D level must be checked by your doctor)
- Vitamin A 25,000 IU
- Zinc 40 mg
- Selenium 200 mcg
- Magnesium 200 to 400 mg
- Quercetin 500 mg
- Garlic 9,000 to 18,000 mg[36]

It is well known that fresh vegetables and fruits are rich in antioxidants to strengthen our immune system. It is important that we stay hydrated with fluids (2,000 ml) to stay physically active to prevent clot formation, to use frequent rest periods, and to preserve energy when extremely tired.

To improve the immune system to be able to fight the virus, daily fresh vegetables high in anti-oxidants (with the power to neutralize free radicals that cause "oxidative stress" which destroys healthy cells, causing inflammation, cancer, heart disease, etc.) are recommended, such as tomatoes, red peppers, garlic, onions, broccoli, kale, red potatoes, spinach, green beans, blueberries, raspberries, strawberries, cranberries, blackberries, oranges, dark chocolate with no sugar, and products that contain probiotics such as plain yogurt, buttermilk, natto, pickles, sauerkraut, kombucha, tempeh, kefir, and other products that are good for a healthy immune system (Dr. Crandall).

CHAPTER 17

Co-Morbidity Prevention

Underlying Conditions

Old people and persons with different medical conditions such as heart disease, diabetes, lung diseases, and those with compromised immune systems are at higher risk to develop serious complications from the disease caused by COVID-19. Dr. Crandall, in Fight Back, emphasizes that "The ISARIC study noted that patients who were hospitalized had certain preexisting conditions, including obesity, heart disease, and diabetes. Such conditions are often associated with the 'metabolic syndrome' that afflicts one-third of adult Americans. People with metabolic syndrome have two or more of the following conditions: obesity, high blood pressure, diabetes, high triglycerides, and low HDL cholesterol, the 'good' cholesterol."[37]

Dr. Blaylock talks about patients with underlying conditions who are at high risk to develop serious symptoms and death, stating, "Only a very small number of people are at risk of a potentially serious outcome from the infection—mainly those with underlying serious medical conditions in conjunction with advanced age and frailty, those with immune compromising conditions, and nursing home patients near the end of their lives. There is growing evidence that the treatment protocol issued to treating doctors by the Centers for Disease Control and Prevention (CDC), mainly intubation and use of a ventilator (respirator), may have contributed significantly to the high death rate in these select individuals."[38]

Know Your Numbers

It is important that we maintain:

- An average blood pressure of 120/80 mmHg for adults (90/60-140/90)
- Blood sugar levels at 70-99 mg/dl before breakfast
- Total cholesterol less than 200 mg/dl
- LDL (bad cholesterol) less than 100 mg/dl
- HDL (good cholesterol) more than 40 mg/dl
- Triglycerides less than 150 mg/dl

Only through lab work ordered by general practitioners can people know the values of their cholesterol, glucose, enzymes, electrolytes, minerals, and vitamin levels. To maintain a normal blood pressure, normal blood sugar level, and normal cholesterol to prevent heart disease and diabetes, it is important every day to follow a healthy diet such as:

- Reduce the consumption of salt with all meals to prevent hypertension. **(It is extremely important to know that during the COVID-19 pandemic, you must check electrolyte levels and blood pressure more frequently, because the virus may reduce sodium levels causing hyponatremia and hypotension, leading to confusion, lethargy, and extreme fatigue. YOU MUST DRINK SALTY LIQUIDS if you get coronavirus symptoms.)**

- Reduce red meat and animal products

- Reduce foods that are greasy such as fats, sauces, cheese, creams, butter, cookies, cakes

- Increase the consumption of vegetables to three to five portions per day

- Increase fruit consumption to two to four portions per day (for diabetes, reduce that to half, one to two portions per day)

- Avoid greasy and oily foods

- Reduce carbohydrates such as potatoes, bread, pasta, rice

- Use sparingly fish oil, avocado, seeds, nuts, olive oil
- Follow a healthy diet with fresh vegetables and fruits
- Reduce consumption of animal proteins, and increase protein consumption from legumes and vegetables such as spinach, peas, soybeans, sprouting broccoli, avocado, beans, garden asparagus, lentil, cauliflower, Brussels sprouts, potatoes, maize, cabbage, artichokes, and others
- Fruits are rich in vitamins, but you must consider the amount of sugar they contain

Obesity is a co-morbidity that causes many complications in patients with COVID-19, leading to death. To reduce body weight and obesity, a person must reduce portions of all foods in order to reduce the amount of calories ingested (except fresh vegetables that are low in calories). The consumption of a low-calorie diet will help a person to reduce weight, which will help to reduce blood pressure and blood sugar levels and lead to better control of hypertension and diabetes.[39]

Intermittent fasting is well documented in literature and helps with our physical and spiritual health. But the Bible gives us many examples of fasting, and guidance for when to engage in intermittent fasting. I cannot stop thinking about biblical examples of people fasting for their spiritual battles and having secondary benefits for their physical health. One example is Daniel fasting, which means to eat only fruits and vegetables for twenty-one days. "In those days I, Daniel, was mourning three full weeks. I ate no pleasant food, no meat or wine came into my mouth, nor did I anoint myself at all, till three whole weeks were fulfilled" (Daniel 10:2-3 NKJV). Daniel had experience with eating vegetables since he had moved into the king's house. "So Daniel said to the steward whom the chief of the eunuchs had set over Daniel, Hananiah, Mishael, and Azariah, 'Please test your servants for ten days, and let them give us vegetables to eat and water to drink...' And at the end of ten days their features appeared better and fatter in flesh than all the young men who ate the portion of the king's delicacies. Thus the steward took away their portion of delicacies and the wine that they were to drink, and gave them vegetables" (Daniel 1:11-16 NKJV). Read the entire book of Daniel to see the benefits of his fasting. I did talk more about that in my first book, Find Your Peace. However, before you decide to fast, talk to your doctor about all your conditions and consult with specialists to see if fasting is for you if you have any health conditions. The sooner the better—then you will know what kind of intermittent fasting you can do to improve your immune system, besides getting strong spiritually.

Dr. Scott Hannen emphasized that regular exercise of about 10,000 steps daily will improve the immune system.[40]

Hydration is very important during this time when fighting COVID-19 with Pedialyte (total fluids per day 2000 ml, which equals 8 glasses of liquids per day, 240 ml each glass).

Follow medical advice from certified medical providers, primary care practitioners, doctors, physicians, nurse practitioners, or general practitioners for any health decision regarding supplements, vitamins, nutrition supplements, type of exercise, any medication, any treatment, any diagnosis, and any medical interventions and procedures:

- Exercise and physical activity every day—at least 10,000 steps or 60-90 minutes a day
- Avoid sedentary life
- Avoid smoking
- Avoid alcohol intake
- Use stress management procedures
- Follow medical advice from your doctor for treatment for diseases that aggravate complications produced by COVID-19 and post COVID-19 symptoms

CHAPTER 18

Post Covid-19

Long-Term Symptoms

Judy George, in her article "80% of COVID-19 Patients May Have Lingering Symptoms, Signs— More Than 50 Effects Persisted After Acute Infection, Meta-analysis Shows" stated,

"'We estimated that a total of 80 percent of the patients infected with SARS-CoV-2 developed one or more long-term symptoms,' Villapol said. 'Preventive measures, rehabilitation techniques, and clinical management strategies designed to address prevalent long-term effects of COVID-19 are urgently needed,' she told *MedPage Today*.

"To date, there's no established diagnosis for the slow, persistent condition that people with lasting effects of COVID-19 experience; terms like 'long COVID,' 'long-haulers,' and 'post-acute COVID-19' have been used, Villapol and colleagues noted. In their review, they referred to lingering symptoms and signs as 'long-term effects of COVID-19.'"[41]

After a few months of the pandemic, we had no information in primary care to guide our practice for post-acute COVID-19 symptoms and what to expect from patients who had recovered from COVID-19. As time passed, we gained some insight as we started to hear from many patients (who had started interventions and treatments in the second week of symptoms) that some symptoms persisted three to four weeks after recovery, or even longer. Some patients who had COVID-19 symptoms after their COVID-19 infection were asking why some symptoms were still present for weeks or months after the COVID-19 season was over, such as dry or wet cough, perspiration, fatigue and getting tired after small tasks, shortness of breath upon exertion, and needing to rest often between tasks. In many cases the patients reported intermittent chest tightness even two months after the virus was gone. It seems like the recovery is very slow.

"Overall, approximately 10% of people who've had COVID-19 experience prolonged symptoms, a UK team estimated in a recently published Practice Pointer on post-acute COVID-19 management. And yet, the authors wrote, primary care physicians have little evidence to guide their care."[42]

Post-COVID Health Conditions

The CDC reported about post COVID-19 health conditions:

As the pandemic unfolds, we are learning that many organs besides the lungs are affected by COVID-19 and there are many ways the infection can affect someone's health. While most persons with COVID-19 recover and return to normal health, some patients can have symptoms that can last for weeks or even months after recovery from acute illness. Even people who are not hospitalized and who have mild illness can experience persistent or late symptoms. Multi-year studies are underway to further investigate. CDC continues to work to identify how common these symptoms are, who is most likely to get them, and whether these symptoms eventually resolve. The most commonly reported long-term symptoms include:

- Fatigue
- Shortness of breath
- Cough
- Joint pain
- Chest pain

Other reported long-term symptoms include:
- Difficulty with thinking and concentration (sometimes referred to as "brain fog")
- Depression
- Muscle pain
- Headache
- Intermittent fever

- Fast-beating or pounding heart (also known as heart palpitations)

More serious long-term complications appear to be less common but have been reported. These have been noted to affect different organ systems in the body. These include:

- Cardiovascular: inflammation of the heart muscle
- Respiratory: lung function abnormalities
- Renal: acute kidney injury
- Dermatologic: rash, hair loss
- Neurological: smell and taste problems, sleep issues, difficulty with concentration, memory problems
- Psychiatric: depression, anxiety, changes in mood[43]

We learned from COVID-19 patients that post CO-VID-19 symptoms are real, and need close monitoring and frequent follow-up visits to provide reassurance, encouragement, and sometimes more treatment, assessment, and evaluation by different specialists such as a cardiologist, pulmonologist, neurologist, nephrologist, endocrinologist, and other specialists as necessary.

CHAPTER 19

Use Both Vaccination and Treatment

Vaccination

"Every good gift and every perfect gift is from above, and cometh down from the Father of lights, with whom is no variableness, neither shadow of turning" (James 1:17, KJV).

I have heard many concerns about vaccines, going from one extreme to the other. The most-asked questions at this time about the vaccine are "What does the vaccine contain?" and "What is it made of?" Here is some very simple information about the ingredients contained in the Pfizer vaccine:

"WHAT ARE THE INGREDIENTS IN THE PFIZ-ER-BIONTECH COVID-19 VACCINE? The Pfizer-BioNTech COVID-19 Vaccine includes the following ingredients: mRNA, lipids ((4-hydroxybutyl)azanediyl) bis(hexane-6,1-diyl)bis(2-hexyldecanoate), 2 [(poly-ethylene glycol)-2000]-N,N-ditetradecylacetamide, 1,2-Distearoyl-sn-glycero-3phosphocholine, and cholesterol), potassium chloride, monobasic potassium phosphate, sodium chloride, dibasic sodium phosphate dihydrate, and sucrose."[44]

COVID-19 mRNA vaccines use a novel approach by which mRNA is delivered into our cells to provide the genetic instructions for our own cells to temporarily make a specific viral protein that triggers an immune response.

Scientists answer the question about the vaccine's ingredients, presenting a simple breakdown of the COVID-19 vaccine as stated here: "The Pfizer-BioNTech COVID-19 vaccine is made of the following ingredients: **mRNA** – Also known as messenger ribonucleic acid, mRNA is the only active ingredient in the vaccine. The mRNA molecules contain the genetic material that provides instructions for our body on how to make a viral protein that triggers an immune response within our bodies. The immune response is what causes our bodies to make the antibodies needed to protect us from getting infected if exposed to the coronavirus. There are rumors that mRNA vaccines will alter our DNA because the RNA molecule can convert information stored in DNA into proteins. That's simply not true. It's critical to note that the mRNA vaccines never enter the nucleus of the cell, where our DNA is stored. After injection, the mRNA from the vaccine is released into the cytoplasm of the cells. Once the viral protein is made and on the surface of the cell, mRNA is broken down and the body permanently gets rid of it, therefore making it impossible to change our DNA."[45]

Pfizer and many pharmaceutical companies have developed vaccines for COVID-19. But even with the 95 percent efficacy demonstrated during trials done by Pfizer, the questions still remain about the duration of immunity created by the anti-COVID-19 vaccine, as Dr. Dormitzer stated in an interview with Serena Marshall on *MedPage Today*: "There'll be many more questions about what is the duration of immunity. Do we start to see cases that're breaking through a long time out? Now, if we were to completely suppress circulation of this virus, well, there'll be no virus circulating to make people sick, but we don't know whether that's the case or not. It is possible. There will still be virus circulating in a significant degree in two years. Or that may not be the case, but regardless, we do want to see how long immunity does last, to the degree that the natural circulation of the virus allows us to do that."[46]

I arrived at the conclusion that we must use precautions to have both the vaccine and the treatment available, during the pandemic and after the pandemic, in the same way we approach other diseases caused by different viruses. For example, for influenza we have both the vaccine and the treatment. A few years ago in our memory care, we had an outbreak of influenza A. We had two confirmed cases, and in order to prevent the spread of influenza to the entire facility we administered the flu vaccine to every person to immunize all the residents. But even with the vaccines people were still getting very sick, and we administered the treatment for influenza even prophylactically to everybody in spite of the vaccine, in order not to let people suffer or die. But despite all of our timely interventions to our elderly people, some of them still passed away in a short time from pneumonia—being frail, old, and having many disabilities for years. From this very simple example we can learn that we need to be more aggressive in treating people early at home if they get sick from the virus, even though they can get a vaccine with high effectiveness. We must be prepared in primary care to intervene early when people get symptoms from the virus, even with vaccination—especially since new mutations happen to viruses every year.

Multiple Vaccines

In my conversation with my friend Dr. Simona Dehelean from San Antonio, Texas, she stated, "We learned that there are several vaccines using different technologies to accomplish the same goal: immunity to COVID-19:

- there are two mRNA (new technology never before used in vaccines) COVID-19 vaccines (by Pfizer and Moderna)
- also, there are two traditional COVID-19 vaccines using an actual COVID-19 protein that is injected into our bodies (made by Novavax and Sanofi-Glaxo-Smith-Kline)
- lastly, also two companies are producing a vaccine that introduces a coronavirus gene to the body using a genetically engineered common-cold virus. This is called a viral vector vaccine (made by AstraZeneca and Johnson & Johnson)."[47]

I did post this information on social media a while ago to answer many questions that people had asked me in private, expressing fear of the unknown about the content and mode of action of the vaccine for CO-VID-19. My answer was: "Fear not the most powerful of God's prescriptions for all humanity to manage stress." This vaccine contains mRNA (enveloped in lipid nanoparticles in a vaccine that is delivered via injection) with genetic instructions for our own cells to produce temporary, specific viral proteins, to trigger our immune systems to produce antibodies to fight the

COVID-19 virus when we are exposed. The Pfizer vaccine does not contain tissues from aborted babies, and does not contain the active or inactive COVID-19 virus. The mRNA does not get into the nucleus of the cells where our DNA resides. It does not affect our DNA. The mRNA disintegrates in about one week and disappears after we develop the antibodies necessary to protect our bodies from the virus.[48]

During my research for more info about the vaccine, I found out that the concept of nanotechnology is not new, and that the vaccines use lipid nanoparticles that "are a vital component of the new Pfizer/BioNTech and Moderna mRNA COVID-19 vaccines, playing a key role in protecting and transporting the mRNA effectively to the right place in the cells... and have been used in numerous clinical trials for anticancer, anti-inflammatory, antibiotic, antifungal, and anaesthetic drug delivery, as well as for the delivery of gene therapies."[49] The reason we get two separate doses is because that will allow time for our body to develop antibodies after the first dose, and then the second dose will give a boost to increase the level of antibodies. What we do not know is how much immunity we will get, and for how long.

Talk to your family doctor and do your own research about vaccination, and make your own decision. We cannot be ignorant of information that is available for early intervention, prophylactic treatment, and vaccination, for physical and spiritual conditions. We must have an understanding of why we take the medications or the vaccines.

I was reflecting on our spiritual condition when we take communion in the remembrance of our LORD Jesus Christ, who died on the cross for the sins of the world and rose again on the third day. We are advised by the Word of God to examine ourselves and be well-informed about our spiritual health and condition, as written in 1 Corinthians 11:28-31 (NIV): "Everyone ought to examine themselves before they eat of the bread and drink from the cup. For those who eat and drink without discerning the body of Christ eat and drink judgment on themselves. That is why many among you are weak and sick, and a number of you have fallen asleep. But if we were more discerning with regard to ourselves, we would not come under such judgment."

PART III

CHAPTER 20

The Treatment for the Soul

Early Interventions for the Soul

"Confess your trespasses to one another, and pray for one another, that you may be healed. The effective, fervent prayer of a righteous man avails much" (James 5:16 NKJV).

As in every physical disease and health condition when we are in emotional distress, besides prevention, early intervention is the key. We have learned from anxiety, depression, and suicide that the treatment for the soul is as important as the treatment for the body. If we treat only the body, the treatment is not complete. When patients with symptoms of the COVID-19 virus were calling me on the phone, I could sense the distress and agony in their soul and in their spirit by the tone of their voices. The "virus of sin" is also an "invisible enemy" for the soul and spirit, infecting the entire world since creation. The world is in turmoil because of the COVID-19 virus but ignores the "virus of sin," with eternal consequences. The antidote is the blood of the Lamb that came to rescue the world from the eternal death caused by sin. My heart was touched by many patients with their physical and emotional pain and suffering. Every single patient expressed concerns and sadness due to the symptoms from the unpredictable virus, to the point of crying and panicking from fear of the disease and death.

As a Christian, I knew that medical treatment was not enough for patients' symptoms in the body, because those symptoms create emotional discomfort. In my spirit I felt their deep pain, and automatically I started to pray fervently for a touch from heaven in their body, soul, and spirit. This verse from James 5:16 resounded in my ears with every sick patient: "Confess your trespasses to one another, and pray for one another, that you may be healed. The effective, fervent prayer of a righteous man avails much" (James 5:16 NKJV).

Prayers Remove the Burden of Fear

Each time I prayed with the patients, I recognized that "the burden of fear" was lifted away at the end of our prayer. I could hear in their voices that the prayer was the "treatment for the soul" that they needed as much as the prescribed medications. I thought to myself that there must be something more, beyond science, to be able to help those in psychological distress from these scary symptoms and diseases caused by the COVID-19 virus that put so much fear in people's minds, affecting their emotions and their quality of life. COVID-19 is a disease that steals the joy from people of all ages.

Prayer is needed, not only to practice our faith. Scientists have demonstrated that prayer and meditation produce significant reductions in blood pressure and heart rate; synchronize breathing and circulation; improve melatonin and serotonin levels; improve the immune system to fight infections from viruses and bacteria; reduce anti-oxidation; reduce stress; promote good moods; and reduce anxiety and pain in degenerative diseases.[50]

When we pray with our patients (who agree with us to pray for them), their emotions are touched by our love for them that medications alone cannot do. They realize that we do not trust only the medications we prescribe, but we trust the One who gives insights to the scientists to develop those medications, and His love is extended to us all. When we pray, the patients feel that we extend our care beyond science to care not only for the body, but for the soul and spirit. We show the love of Jesus in providing holistic care with love that is unconditional.

COVID-19 AND POST COVID-19 ALLEVIATE THE FEAR

Give Unconditional Love

William A. Petri, Jr., MD, PhD, Professor of Medicine in the Division of Infectious Diseases & International Health at the University of Virginia, Vice Chair of the Department of Medicine, stated in "Prayer from the Front Lines of Coronavirus Research" on March 14, 2020, "In my position, the only approach to working with someone else is to give them unconditional love. That's what was given to me by Christ, dying on the cross for me. If you're giving someone unconditional love, it is so freeing. If this person says something that irritates you, that slight doesn't matter because this is all about, 'What can I contribute for this person?'"[51]

For me, when patients with signs and symptoms of the COVID-19 virus called, and after I discussed their condition in detail and the plan for treatment, I asked them if they would let me pray for them. There are two reason why I offer prayer: 1) my heart is broken for their physical and emotional suffering, and 2) I am in desperation for them, because of the virus' unknown mechanism of actions and unpredictable progression—destroying cells, tissues, systems, and organs, leading to long-term consequences for some patients, and for others leading to multiple trips to the ER, hospitalization, complications, ventilators, and in some cases death—and medical providers are hopeless and helpless at this point.

Many times, during my prayer time with the patients by phone, I heard the patient sobbing or crying, pouring her/his heart to God. One patient, crying, stated, "That is what I needed: prayer." Prayer in the name of Jesus Christ is a part of the early intervention.

I heard many testimonies from patients of how the prayer helped them with their symptoms. One patient (V), who had prolonged symptoms of extreme fatigue and weakness, stated, "The healing process started when we prayed on the phone." Three other patients (A, G, and L) were in desperation that their fever had not subsided for more than a week, even though they were taking "lots" of Tylenol. They stated that the fever stopped after we prayed. When I followed up, the patients stated that they were doing well—the medications had helped in two to three days, but "the prayer helped them right away." Another patient reported that his heart rate had normalized on the day we prayed on the phone for a normal heart rate.

Dr. Scott Hannen, in his book *Stop the Pain*, stated that we can find fifteen minutes to pause and pray to reduce the stress that causes inflammation and damage to the organs in our body (page 271).[52]

Improve Immunity through Prayer

We know very well now that COVID-19 causes anywhere from mild to severe inflammation to the organs in the body due to a weak immune system that over-reacts and does not work properly. It is well documented in literature that prayer helps our immune system to get stronger through the healthy neurochemicals released in our body when we focus on the things of God—the source of our health, our Creator. Increased fear suppresses humans' immunity, but prayer enhances its effectiveness. Prayer is tight to healing. Healing depends on prayer. When I pray in desperation with patients, I make a statement and pray that the medication I prescribe will do the job that it is supposed to do, but healing comes from God. The Bible says that when the Israelites were sick with many diseases, God sent His Word to heal them, as written in Psalm 107:20-22. "He sent His word and healed them, and delivered them from their destructions. Oh, that men would give thanks to the LORD for His goodness, and for His wonderful works to the children of men! Let them sacrifice the sacrifices of thanksgiving, and declare His works with rejoicing" (Psalm 107:20-22 NKJV). God's Word is God's prescription for health and has the power to heal our physical and spiritual diseases.

I obeyed the Holy Spirit and I did pray fervently throughout the day for every single patient who I knew was sick. I heard patients giving testimonies after prayers when I followed up daily on their conditions—how their symptoms improved and their joy was restored. Staying in touch with each patient, texting or calling them every day, gave them so much relief from the fear of the diseases caused by the virus. I decided to trust God in caring for our patients. I remember how I had held my faith very strong during the communist regime in Romania. How much more here, in a country built on Judeo-Christian faith, values, and beliefs.

Holistic care is the key to addressing the entire person's needs—physically, mentally, spiritually, and socially. Emotions are real factors that contribute to the well-being of a person. I observed firsthand, day by day, how patients responded to my checking on them with my daily follow-up and prayer, giving them hope in God's promises for divine health and complete healing. By reading my texts or hearing my voice on the phone, hope was aroused in their minds and hearts and changed their emotional states. I could hear the calmness in their voices and expressions of hope. I made it a habit to text them a verse from the Bible—the Living Word of God—or encouraging, positive words with God's promises, to increase their faith and to decrease fear. Faith is antidote for fear.

God's Mystery—Prayer

Prayer is the most powerful tool in any circumstances. I used to tell people that prayer is God's mystery, for every human being to enter into His spiritual realm and connect with His supernatural power for supernatural intervention in every human's life. He gave us the command to pray, not to understand prayer. Our Creator wants us to communicate with Him. "Then Aaron took it as Moses commanded, and ran into the midst of the assembly; and already the plague had begun among the people. So he put in the incense and made atonement for the people. And he stood between the dead and the living; so the plague was stopped" (Numbers 16:47-48 NKJV). The incense means the prayers—according to the Word of God, according to Revelation 5:8 (NKJV): "Now when he had taken the scroll, the four living creatures and the twenty-four elders fell down before the Lamb, each having a harp, and golden bowls full of incense, which are the prayers of the saints."

Prayer in Christ's name is the most important part of treatment. Dr. Crandall, MD, cardiologist, director of the largest program of heart transplants in the world, stated that in medicine we must give people "the best of medicine and the best of Christ."

By faith in prayer, we can ask God to intervene on our behalf even during this pandemic situation. I am convinced that God has intervened and spared many lives in the USA during the COVID-19 pandemic.

"The White House models they displayed showed that more than 2.2 million people could have died in the United States if nothing were done." I believe that millions of people around the world prayed, and God intervened and spared the population of the USA and the earth.[53]

C.H. Spurgeon stated in his book *Prayer*: "We want to draw near to You now through Jesus Christ the Mediator, and we want to be bold to speak to You as a man speaks with his friend. Have You not said by Your Spirit, 'Let us therefore come boldly unto the throne of grace' (Hebrews 4:16)?"[54]

CHAPTER 21

Hope, the Anchor of the Soul

Manage Stress from COVID-19 by Activating Hope

This is a time when you cannot afford to live a stressful life. Diseases, pain, and disabilities are real, and death is real. They put into our minds tormenting thoughts of fear that affect our body, soul, and spirit. I approach patients as real people with a body, soul, and spirit, and I try to be fair in all approaches to address people's needs with the truth in my heart and mind as my Creator cares for me. He is the One who brings healing and comfort and restores joy in my life. That increases my faith and my hope, which further reduces stress. Isaiah reassures us that God sent Jesus Christ, His Son, "To console those who mourn in Zion, to give them beauty for ashes, the oil of joy for mourning, the garment of praise for the spirit of heaviness; that they may be called trees of righteousness, the planting of the LORD, that He may be glorified" (Isaiah 61:3 NKJV).

I like research, and the best scientific evidence and results, but I must acknowledge the limitations I see in our capabilities to control pandemics—with consequences for the entire world—even with the highest expertise and the most advanced technology. We do not have a 100 percent guarantee in any disease, with our skills, knowledge, and expertise—even though they make a huge difference in people's lives—that we can trust that we will have 100 percent control. After thirty years in the long-term care business, I can make this statement: More research is needed in every area of human suffering. I have seen patients with fifteen to twenty different medications on their lists who still continued to suffer from their chronic diseases and disabilities, and who finally died from those diseases. The only hope someone can have is in Jesus Christ, who saves our being and anchors our soul to God's power and presence. It is written in Hebrews 6:19 that "This hope we have as an anchor of the soul, both sure and steadfast, and which enters the Presence behind the veil" (Hebrews 6:19 NKJV).

When we believe in our heart that Jesus Christ is the Son of God, who died on the cross for our sins and shed His blood to save the world; and that God did raise Him from the dead; and we confess with our mouth that He is Lord over our life, opening our heart and letting Him take residence in us through the power of the Holy

Spirit; He becomes our hope of glory, as stated in Colossians 1:27. "To them God willed to make known what are the riches of the glory of this mystery among the Gentiles: which is Christ in you, the hope of glory" (Colossians 1:27 NKJV).

Hope in God's Supernatural Wisdom

Without hope in God's supernatural power, all efforts, using physical and intellectual resources, that we make to prevent the spread of the virus and to prescribe treatments are limited; we must recognize that we cannot trust in our own wisdom, knowledge, and understanding during a pandemic time. We have proved that we are incompetent to prevent disaster in the world in the face of this virus—the cruel enemy of our body, soul, and spirit—physically, emotionally, socially, economically, ethically, etc. In Proverbs 3:5-6 we read, "Trust in the LORD with all your heart, and lean not on your own understanding; in all your ways acknowledge Him, and He shall direct your paths" (Proverbs 3:5-6 NKJV).

Hope increases when we acknowledge God's supernatural wisdom in every discovery we make through research and recognize that every gift is from Him through the Holy Spirit, who is real and at work on this planet according to James 1:17. "Every good gift and every perfect gift is from above, and comes down from the Father of lights, with whom there is no variation or shadow of turning" (James 1:17 NKJV). We did not bring anything into this world. Our capability to design studies, and for understanding and interpreting the results from science, and our ability to memorize and remember information is from our Creator, Jehovah Elohim, the Creator of the heavens and earth. Through the power of the Holy Spirit, we receive wisdom and inspiration and discernment and become knowledgeable in our world to function as we do through our actions.

Everything we know—I mean everything on this planet since its creation—is from God the Father through His precious Son Jesus Christ, as is written in Ephesians 1:17-19: "That the God of our Lord Jesus Christ, the Father of glory, may give to you the spirit of wisdom and revelation in the knowledge of Him, the eyes of your understanding being enlightened; that you may know what is the hope of His calling, what are the riches of the glory of His inheritance in the saints, and what is the exceeding greatness of His power toward us who believe, according to the working of His mighty power" (Ephesians 1:17-19 NKJV).

God's Promises for Healing

"For I am the LORD who heals you" (Exodus 15:26 NKJV).

The key to being healed is to listen diligently to God's voice and obey by doing what is right in His sight. In Exodus 15:26 God promised, "If you diligently heed the voice of the LORD your God and do what is right in His sight, give ear to His commandments and keep all His statutes, I will put none of the diseases on you which I have brought on the Egyptians. For I am the LORD who heals you" (Exodus 15:26 NKJV).

Trust the Word of God and have faith in Jesus Crist. He is moved with compassion and wants to heal every suffering person when we come to Him with childlike faith. The Bible tells us that "Jesus went through all the towns and villages, teaching in their synagogues, proclaiming the good news of the kingdom and healing every disease and sickness. When he saw the crowds, he had compassion on them, because they were harassed and helpless, like sheep without a shepherd" (Mathew 9:35-36 NIV).

Jesus died on the cross for our sins, so that our souls can be saved through His suffering and His wounds, to receive healing. The prophet Isaiah wrote in chapter 53 verse 5, "But he was pierced for our transgressions, he was crushed for our iniquities; the punishment that brought us peace was on him, and by his wounds we are healed" (Isaiah 53:5 NIV).

When we seek God's forgiveness for all our sins, He is faithful to forgive all our sins and to heal our diseases.

"Praise the Lord, my soul; all my inmost being, praise his holy name. Praise the Lord, my soul, and forget not all his benefits—who forgives all your sins and heals all your diseases" (Psalm 103:1-3 NIV). Forgiveness of our sins is the key to healing for all our diseases to come.

Divine Protection in the Shadow of His Wings

As a health care professional for three decades, and as a general practitioner providing direct care to thousands of patients with acute and chronic illnesses to the end of their lives and seeing them dying over the years, I know that we have only one hope in God and His Son Jesus' blood to cover us and to protect us in the shadow of His wings—as is written in Psalm 91, which I have often used to encourage myself when I have gone through struggles in my life. I echo Mr. Stephen Strang, who stated in his book *God, Trump, and COVID-19: How the Pandemic Is Affecting Christians, the World, and America's 2020 Election,* that "I believe strongly that God has given us a powerful and miraculous immune system to fight off the possible trillions of viruses in the world. Many of today's processed foods and GMOs directly target our immune system. This only solidifies the case to build our immunity and practice wisdom in our eating habits. Dr. Colbert told me that, first of all, as Christians we must approach this pandemic with faith and not fear. We must pray Psalm 91 over ourselves and our families:

'Surely He shall deliver you from the snare of the hunter and from the deadly pestilence' (Ps. 91:3 MEV). 'Read the Word out loud over yourself and your family every day, and then receive that word by faith and don't live in fear,' Colbert said. I would add that we should plead the blood of Jesus over ourselves and our loved ones each day and truly put on the full armor of God. After all, in many ways this is what we have trained for."[55]

From my experience as a Christian who lived in a communist country for more than three decades and a strong believer in God's Word, I can strongly encourage patients to pray boldly: "Keep me as the apple of Your eye; hide me under the shadow of Your wings" (Psalm 17:8 NKJV), and: "I will say of the LORD, 'He is my refuge and my fortress; My God, in Him I will trust'" (Psalm 91:2 NKJV).

As we practice social distancing, we can get near to God in His spiritual realm through prayers, and as we wear masks, we can raise our voices to our God in the Holy Spirit, getting closer to our Creator.

I am sharing with you, the readers, so you know that the battle is not against flesh but against principalities. "For we do not wrestle against flesh and blood, but against principalities, against powers, against the rulers of the darkness of this age, against spiritual hosts of wickedness in the heavenly places" (Ephesians 6:12 NKJV). Fear is the enemy of our body, soul, and spirit.

Because all things shall pass away, we must be people waiting for the Lord to return in faith.

Church is Essential for Physical and Spiritual Healing

Church is a place where people worship God, the Creator of the universe, together in the Spirit—a place where people of faith fellowship and have a sense of belonging, where their spiritual needs are satisfied and the joy of the Lord is restored in their soul. For their physical and spiritual health, people need to communicate and to interact with each other, socialize, and get support. A church is a "spiritual clinic" where people's souls get restored, and emotions are healed when experiencing psychological distress. I am writing in the hope that we the people will learn from our past mistakes and will not close the churches again. Other measures can be implemented. Groups of people can take turns throughout the week, but the church should stay open as the ER is open twenty-four hours a day, seven days a week. God created humans to worship Him. We see throughout the Bible that worship is essential for God to be present in the middle of a congregation. "Then the LORD said to Moses, 'Go to Pharaoh and say to him, "This is what the LORD, the God of the Hebrews, says: 'Let my people go, so that they may worship me'"'" (Exodus 9:1 NIV). God knew that we were created for worship so He could present Himself in our midst. During a pandemic time, the worst thing to do is to close the houses of worship so humans are depleted of God's presence when they need Him the most. As we must have food available for the body, so we must have spiritual food available twenty-four hours a day. With no spiritual food, the soul will die.

CHAPTER 22

Encouragement for Those Who Mourn

He Heals the Brokenhearted

"He heals the brokenhearted and binds up their wounds" (Psalm 147:3 NKJV).

During this pandemic, I have heard as never before news of younger people dying in every corner of this planet. The emotional pain of separation through death is real and unbearable. To be able to bear that emotional pain and avoid depression from prolonged feelings of sadness, one must run to God's Word and fill his/her heart with the Holy Spirit's power, who is able through God's promises to give peace, joy, and hope, according to Romans 15:13. "May the God of hope fill you with all joy and peace in believing, so that by the power of the Holy Spirit you may abound in hope" (Romans 15:13

ESV). God in heaven is the One and Only who can heal the brokenhearted and bind those deep wounds created by the painful separation of death.

We always must have hope in God's promises, that He is breathing the breath of life into us even in the most difficult and impossible circumstances and will make us live, as He did breathe on "dry bones" and made them live, as we read in Ezekiel chapter 37. It is a long passage of Scripture, but it is a powerful illustration of the supernatural power of the Spirit of God who made "dry bones" to become alive. "The hand of the LORD came upon me and brought me out in the Spirit of the LORD, and set me down in the midst of the valley; and it was full of bones. Then He caused me to pass by them all around, and behold, there were very many in the open valley; and indeed they were very dry. And He said to me, 'Son of man, can these bones live?' So I answered, 'O Lord GOD, You know.' Again He said to me, 'Prophesy to these bones, and say to them, "O dry bones, hear the word of the LORD! Thus says the Lord GOD to these bones: 'Surely I will cause breath to enter into you, and you shall live. I will put sinews on you and bring flesh upon you, cover you with skin and put breath in you; and you shall live. Then you shall know that I am the LORD.'"' So I prophesied as I was commanded; and as I prophesied, there was a noise, and suddenly a rattling; and the bones came together, bone to bone. Indeed, as I looked, the sinews and the flesh came upon them, and the skin covered them over; but there was no breath in them. Also He said to me, 'Prophesy to the breath, prophesy, son of man, and say to the breath, "Thus says the Lord GOD: 'Come from the four winds, O breath, and breathe on these slain, that they may live.'"' So I prophesied as He commanded me, and breath came into them, and they lived, and stood upon their feet, an exceedingly great army. Then He said to me, 'Son of man, these bones are the whole house of Israel. They indeed say, "Our bones are dry, our hope is lost, and we ourselves are cut off!" Therefore prophesy and say to them, "Thus says the Lord GOD: 'Behold, O My people, I will open your graves and cause you to come up from your graves, and bring you into the land of Israel. Then you shall know that I am the LORD, when I have opened your graves, O My people, and brought you up from your graves. I will put My Spirit in you, and you shall live, and I will place you in your own land. Then you shall know that I, the LORD, have spoken it and performed it,' says the LORD"'" (Ezekiel 37:1-14 NKJV).

As in ancient times, once again all nations on earth became a "death valley" full of "death bones," because the joy was stolen by the "invisible enemy" that infiltrates every single nation. As I mentioned earlier, it is written in Proverbs 17:12 that "A cheerful heart is good medicine, but a crushed spirit dries up the bones" (Proverbs 17:22 NIV). The entire world is affected by the fear of COVID-19 that has "crushed the spirit" of humanity and caused anxiety and depression, bringing more physical and spiritual diseases and premature death. The joy was gone, leaving the entire world with physical and spiritual consequences. Without joy, the bones of humanity become "dry bones." The spirit of the world is crushed by the fear of COVID-19 which "dries the bones," crippling people's lives.

Breathe Again

Once again, God wants to breathe into us all in order for us to be able to live, physically and spiritually. God's desire is that we know His Holy Spirit of the living God is real, and He can breathe His Spirit on us, His people, and we can live in this land to see the goodness of God in the land of the living—to recognize that HE IS the great "I AM," Jehovah Shamma, God who is present in every moment of our lives to meet our needs. Only a Holy God can restore the joy of our soul that can bring healing and restoration. Without that joy of salvation, nations will continue to "dry up," becoming a "valley of dried bones." Our hearts must be filled with hope, joy, and peace when fear of COVID-19 paralyzes people during a pandemic situation. People are suffering with severe symptoms in our community and do not have a place to go for help, being forced to adopt a "sicken-in-place" paradigm until sick enough—with difficulty breathing and respiratory distress, when oxygen levels drop below the normal range—to be admitted to the hospital and in some cases, to die prematurely. Our spiritual life is affected by fear and increased stress from worries and worldly things, affecting our spiritual breath. The Bible gives us clear instructions and guidance on how to behave in our era, with the most advanced technology, the best experts, and advanced science, with excellence in our daily life. "Finally, brothers, whatever is true, whatever is honorable, whatever is just, whatever is pure, whatever is lovely, whatever is commendable, if there is any excellence, if there is anything worthy of praise, think about these things" (Philippians 4:8 ESV).

God, the Creator of the universe, gave us all things that pertain to life and excellence to help us escape corruption in the world, as is written 2 Peter 1:3-4. "His divine power has granted to us all things that pertain to life and godliness, through the knowledge of him who called us to his own glory and excellence, by which he has granted to us his precious and very great promises, so that through them you may become partakers of the divine nature, having escaped from the corruption that is in the world because of sinful desire" (2 Peter 1:3-4 ESV).

The book of Genesis tells us that we were created in a unique way by God to follow His purpose for our life here on earth. "So God created man in His own image; in the image of God He created him; male and female He created them" (Genesis 1:27 NKJV). Each person is uniquely created, fearfully and wonderfully, by the Creator. In Psalm 139 it is written, "For You formed my inward parts; You covered me in my mother's womb. I will praise You, for I am fearfully and wonderfully made; marvelous are Your works, and that my soul knows very well" (Psalm 139:13-14 NKJV). Because of God's unique purpose in creation, each person is different—even in developing symptoms from diseases caused by the virus—and has a different clinical presentation after contracting the COVID-19 virus because of our uniqueness as God's creation.[56]

So every single person develops different symptoms from this "invisible enemy," trying to fight an unpredictable virus, and needs to be treated as soon as possible and even prescribed prophylactic treatments, as many medical doctors have proved to work to prevent people from dying from the virus. (See all studies and protocols mentioned above, and more are yet to be developed.)

Sin in the world is another "invisible enemy" that produces spiritual diseases.

I have learned over the years as a strong believer in the power of the living Word of God that people are healed physically and spiritually through the best of medicine and the best of Christ, as many Christian doctors and general practitioners have proved in their practices. And when doctors and specialists have no control over a disease and it is beyond their knowledge and expertise, and people are not healed in the body, because of their restored soul and spiritual health they move to their eternal home—prepared by the Lord for those who believe in Him—to glorify the LORD with the cloud of witnesses who are waiting for all of us who remain on earth to join them one day to give glory to our Father for ever and ever and ever.

We are assured by His living Word telling us: "Most assuredly, I say to you, he who hears My word and believes in Him who sent Me has everlasting life, and shall not come into judgment, but has passed from death into life" (John 5:24 NKJV).

CHAPTER 23

Can God Punish Sin?

"The Lord is not slow in keeping his promise, as some understand slowness. Instead he is patient with you, not wanting anyone to perish, but everyone to come to repentance" (2 Peter 3:9 NIV).

God Waits for Everyone to Repent

Many people ask if this virus is a plague that God sent to punish the world for sin. All I can say is that God does punish sin and those who offend His Holy name. He is God. We are not. We are His creation. We must fear God as a person and as a nation. He is a good God, but because He is Holy and cannot tolerate sin, He is also a ferocious God and can punish all nations on earth when they ignore His commandments. He can destroy nations for living in sin and for dishonoring Him and His living Word. He did that in ancient times, and He will do it again to get the entire world's attention. "And don't forget Sodom and Gomorrah and their neighboring towns, which were filled with immorality and every kind of sexual perversion. Those cities were destroyed by fire and serve as a warning of the eternal fire of God's judgment" (Jude 1:7 NLT).

Killing babies in their mothers' wombs upsets God the most, because they are His creation, created in God's image. He gave directions and instructions to the first couple, Adam and Eve, when He created male and female in the Garden of Eden to be fruitful and multiply. That was the purpose for creation. But humans took the matter into their own hands and ignored their Creator's plan and will. Humanity went so far as to kill their own babies. We read in the Old Testament how horrible is the sin of abortion.

"The LORD said to Moses, 'Say to the Israelites: "Any Israelite or any foreigner residing in Israel who sacrifices any of his children to Molek is to be put to death. The members of the community are to stone him. I myself will set my face against him and will cut him off from his people; for by sacrificing his children to Molek, he has defiled my sanctuary and profaned my holy name. If the members of the community close their eyes when that man sacrifices one of his children to Molek and if they fail to put him to death, I myself will set my face against him and his family and will cut them off from their people together with all who follow him in prostituting themselves to Molek. I will set my face against anyone who turns to mediums and spiritists to prostitute themselves by following them, and I will cut them off from their people. Consecrate yourselves and be holy, because I am the LORD your God. Keep my decrees and follow them. I am the LORD, who makes you holy"'" (Leviticus 20:1-8 NIV).

How many babies are killed through abortion in this country and around the world? The answer is tens of millions. You can search for yourselves. Is God upset? Based on the verses in the Bible, yes. He is. But He is waiting patiently that people and nations will return and come to Him in repentance. He does not want anyone to perish. "The Lord is not slow in keeping his promise, as some understand slowness. Instead he is patient with you, not wanting anyone to perish, but everyone to come to repentance" (2 Peter 3:9 NIV). God is Holy and is asking His creation to be holy also. Living in righteousness is God's heart desire for a nation, as it is written in Proverbs 14:34, that "Righteousness exalts a nation, but sin is a reproach to any people" (Proverbs 14:34 NKJV). God calls us to repentance and prayer for the nation and the city where we live in order to live in peace and to prosper, as is written in Jeremiah 29:7. "Also, seek the peace and prosperity of the city to which I have carried you into exile. Pray to the LORD for it, because if it prospers, you too will prosper" (Jeremiah 29:7 NIV).

This is a great opportunity to reassess your relationship with Jesus Christ, the Lamb of God, who died on the cross for the sins of the entire world and rose again on the third day, and who is waiting for every sinner to confess their sins and to receive Him as their personal Savior. Without Jesus Christ there is no salvation from our sins, and no eternal life in heaven, and life on earth has no meaning. Jesus is the only Way to heaven. "Jesus said to him, 'I am the way, the truth, and the life. No one comes to the Father except through Me'" (John 14:6 NKJV).

The only hope is Jesus Christ for our sins to be forgiven and to have eternal life with Him in heaven, after this one on earth passes away. Each one of us needs Jesus Christ to wash our sins away, because we are all sinners, as is written in Romans 3:23-26. "For all have sinned and fall short of the glory of God, being justified freely by His grace through the redemption that is in Christ Jesus, whom God set forth as a propitiation by His blood, through faith, to demonstrate His righteousness, because in His forbearance God had passed over the sins that were previously committed, to demonstrate at the present time His righteousness, that He might be just and the justifier of the one who has faith in Jesus" (Romans 3:23-26 NKJV).

Example of Prayer of Repentance

I am writing this example of a prayer to receive Jesus Christ into your heart, in order for you to receive forgiveness of your sins and to start a new life on earth that will lead to eternal life in heaven, to be with the LORD for ever and ever after this temporary life on this planet is over:

"Father God in heaven, I have sinned against You. I recognize and confess all my sins, from when I was born until today. Please forgive all my sins and wash them away with the precious blood of the Lamb. I bring all my sins to the cross. Cleanse me with the precious holy blood that was shed by the Lamb of God, Your Son, Jesus Christ. Come into my heart through the power of the Holy Spirit and be my personal Lord and Savior. Transform my life. Today I want to start a new life with You, Jesus Christ, who died on the cross for my sins, and was resurrected on the third day and ascended to heaven, and who is sitting at the right hand of God, the Father, the Creator of the universe, to intercede for me, my family, and the entire world. Thank You. In Jesus' name I pray."

That powerful prayer will change your "spiritual DNA" when your thoughts are changed, releasing a healthy amount of neurotransmitters and making you a new creation in Christ Jesus. You will receive unspeakable joy and peace—and no stress from fear caused by COVID-19.[57]

We know that each one of us on earth will die one day and must face God's judgment as, it is written in Hebrews 9:27-28 that "Just as people are destined to die once, and after that to face judgment, so Christ was sacrificed once to take away the sins of many; and he will appear a second time, not to bear sin, but to bring salvation to those who are waiting for him" (Hebrews 9:27-28 NIV)."For he says, 'In the time of my favor I heard you, and in the day of salvation I helped you.' I tell you, now is the time of God's favor, now is the day of salvation" (2 Corinthians 6:2 NIV).

The day we leave this planet is the most important day in each person's life. It is important to be ready for that day, because we do not know when our time will be up to leave this planet. Today is the day to receive God's salvation, when He shows the entire world His favor to receive salvation.

CHAPTER 24

Conclusion

The overwhelming news of COVID-19 started to spread on the local, national, and international news, on TV, the internet, social media, in the newspaper, on the radio, in stores, and at work, and the fear started to escalate. When I talked to family members, neighbors, friends, pastors, doctors, politicians, legislators, lay persons, and professional people in our city, state, country, and abroad, I could sense the sadness that was pinning everyone's thoughts to one word—COVID-19—that would dictate our everyday life for the rest of the year.

I knew exactly the consequences of fear and sadness: stirring up negative thoughts, causing a shift in neurotransmitters and decreasing serotonin, dopamine, endorphins, melatonin, and other neurochemicals, leading to depression and its consequences. The battle is real in our mind through thoughts of fear and despair. Thoughts of fear take up "real estate" in our brain, with billions of neurons and repeating thoughts of fear in our mind—and will control it, causing the immune system to weaken and not be able to fight the COVID-19 virus and causing more damage to our body, soul, and spirit.

I knew that the only way to overcome fear is by faith, which is the uncontestable antidote for every fearful situation, and that faith comes by hearing. I knew from my own experience that only the living Word of God can help to banish fear, reassuring us that He is with us in the most difficult time. "And the LORD, He is the One who goes before you. He will be with you, He will not leave you nor forsake you; do not fear nor be dismayed" (Deuteronomy 31:8 NKJV).

After almost thirty years of providing end-of-life care for elderly people with multiple chronic conditions (and as a general practitioner in primary care), just three months before the pandemic I was led miraculously by the Holy Spirit to a very small health clinic, a place where patients (minorities) were able to receive care with the love of Christ in such as time as this. A place where I could volunteer my time, with a mission to prevent diseases and to restore joy by promoting health physically, emotionally, and spiritually. Joy is one of the most powerful emotions that brings healing to our body, spirit, and soul.

Joy is the antidote for sadness and depression. The reward mechanism in our brain is activated when we are full of joy and dopamine is released, improving our motivation for the activities of daily living and everyday life. Serotonin and endorphins, oxytocin, and other neurochemicals are released in the body to restore our health and to keep us healthy and motivated to move on with life.

To dissipate thoughts of fear and sadness during a pandemic is extremely difficult, especially when patients and their families are facing an aggressive virus, an "invisible enemy," with symptoms that have led to millions of deaths in the world. I reviewed thoroughly the information with the protocols and the algorithms for early interventions at home developed by top doctors, experts, and researchers such as the one published in the Journal of *American Medicine* by et. al., who emphasized in the article "Pathophysiological Basis and Rationale for Early Outpatient Treatment of SARS-CoV-2 (COVID-19) Infection" that "Therapeutic approaches based on these principles include 1) reduction of reinoculation, 2) combination antiviral therapy, 3) immunomodulation, 4) antiplatelet/antithrombotic therapy, and 5) administration of oxygen, monitoring, and telemedicine."[58]

Throughout this pandemic, people have had endless questions due to the unknowns and uncertainties they face. We direct them to the resources available and to professional health care providers, doctors, and nurses working in the health field who are knowledgeable and up to date, informing people of how to get relief from their fear, anxiety, and depression. The CDC displays all of these recommendations on the internet, easily accessible by any person.

We can have peace that passes all understanding when we get wisdom from above during this hard time through the pandemic. "He who gets wisdom loves his own soul; he who keeps understanding will find good" (Proverbs 19:8 NKJV).

This is a time when we cannot afford to live a stressful life. Diseases, pain, and disabilities are real, and death is real. They put into our minds tormenting thoughts of fear that affect our body, soul, and spirit. I approach patients as real people with a body, soul, and spirit, and I try to be fair in all approaches to address people's needs with the truth in my heart and mind as my Creator cares for me. He is the One who brings healing and comfort and restores joy in my life. That increases my faith and my hope, which further reduces stress. Isaiah reassures us that God sent Jesus Christ, His Son, "to console those who mourn in Zion, to give them beauty for ashes, the oil of joy for mourning, the garment of praise for the spirit of heaviness; that they may be called trees of righteousness, the planting of the LORD, that He may be glorified" (Isaiah 61:3 NKJV).

"For I am the LORD who heals you" (Exodus 15:26 NKJV).

The key to being healed is to listen diligently to God's voice and obey by doing what is right in His sight. In Exodus 15:26 God promised, "If you diligently heed the voice of the LORD your God and do what is right in His sight, give ear to His commandments and keep all His statutes, I will put none of the diseases on you which I have brought on the Egyptians. For I am the LORD who heals you" (Exodus 15:26 NKJV).

The Holy Spirit prompted me to share my experience and my patients' stories that we may get insights if another pandemic is coming, or for any difficult situation in our lives. We all learn from mistakes sometimes in life, when we go through uncertain and unknown circumstances. We cannot be ignorant of our experience in the past and the knowledge and resources available at a crucial moment to get over and to move on with life on this planet.

About the Author

Born in Romania in a large family of eight siblings, Rodica Malos's family suffered under communist tyranny and oppression because of their strong Christian beliefs. Yet Rodica has never lost her faith in the power of the Word of God, especially its ability to promote physical and spiritual health. Growing up in impoverished conditions and facing constant opposition because of her faith, Rodica persevered and, through hard work, achieved a high level of education. After graduating from the Academy of Economic Science in Bucharest, she worked as an economist for a large company until leaving the country. Arriving in the United States in 1990 with no English skills or finances, initially, she earned a living doing janitorial work and as a caregiver for elderly nursing home patients. Thanks to saving and carefully budgeting her money, in 1992, she launched an at-home business offering foster care. Rodica also enrolled in health nursing and medical studies and eventually earned several degrees, including doctor of nursing practice from Oregon Health & Science University (OHSU). Rodica worked in the health care field for about three decades. She and her husband, Stelica, as the founders and operators of Malos Adult Foster Homes, Tabor Crest Residential Care (memory care), and Tabor Crest II Memory Care provided physical, emotional, and spiritual care (including comfort care at the end of life) to elderly patients with multiple chronic conditions, including neurocognitive disorders and memory loss. Since 1997, Dr. Malos has volunteered more than five thousand hours of her time to help the less fortunate. She has served as a registered nurse in community care and as a primary care provider at

Portland Adventist Community Service Health Clinic. With Agape Health Care, she has provided care for minorities and others lacking access to the health care system. She also organizes health fairs and free clinics in Portland and other countries. Currently, Dr. Malos is working as a general practitioner/primary care provider at a Community Health Clinic in Portland, Oregon. Married to Stelica since 1986, she and her husband have one daughter, Andreea, who also graduated from OHSU with a doctor of pharmacy degree. Also, Dr. Rodica is an international speaker and organizes and speaks at medical and spiritual Christian conferences in USA and abroad. As a board member at Star of Hope International, she travels abroad and supports children with disabilities and their families financially, emotionally, and spiritually. She is the author of *Find Your Peace: Supernatural Solutions Beyond Science for Fear, Anxiety, and Depression* and *Created in His Image with Unique Purpose (Science and Beyond)*. Holy Spirit is Real. Her website is http://www.rodicamalos.com.

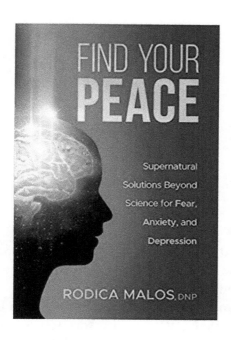

FIND YOUR **PEACE**

Supernatural Solutions Beyond Science for Fear, Anxiety, and Depression

RODICA MALOS, DNP

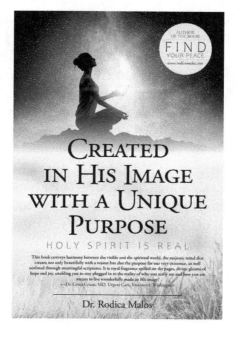

AUTHOR OF THE BOOK

FIND YOUR PEACE
www.rodicamalos.com

CREATED IN HIS IMAGE WITH A UNIQUE PURPOSE

HOLY SPIRIT IS REAL

This book conveys harmony between the visible and the spiritual world, the majestic mind that creates not only beautifully with a reason but also the purpose for our very existence, so well outlined through meaningful scriptures. It is royal fragrance spilled on the pages, divine gleams of hope and joy, enabling you to stay plugged in to the reality of who you really are and how you are meant to live wonderfully made in *His image!*
—Dr. Crina Crisan, MD, Urgent Care, Vancouver, Washington

Dr. Rodica Malos

Endnotes

1 Dr. David Levy. Fear in Crisis - Part 1 (Help for Coronavirus COVID-19): Overcoming Anxiety. YouTube. Accessed Nov. 20, 2020.

2 Mary Van Beusekom. Depression triples in US adults amid COVID-19 stressors. CIDRAP. Sep 03, 2020. https://www.cidrap.umn.edu/news-perspective/2020/09/depression-triples-us-adults-amid-covid-19-stressors. Accessed Nov. 1, 2020.

3 Czeisler, MÉ, Lane, RI, Petrosky, E, et. al. Mental Health, Substance Use, and Suicidal Ideation During the COVID-19 Pandemic — United States, June 24–30, 2020. MMWR Morb Mortal Wkly Rep 2020;69:1049–1057. DOI: http://dx.doi.org/10.15585/mmwr.mm6932a1. https://www.cdc.gov/mmwr/volumes/69/wr/mm6932a1.htm. Accessed Nov. 1, 2020.

4 Peter A. McCullough, MD, MPH. . Pathophysiological Basis and Rationale for Early Outpatient Treatment of SARS-CoV-2 (COVID-19) Infection. The American Journal of Medicine, 7 August 2020. https://www.sciencedirect.com/science/article/pii/S0002934320306732. Accessed Nov. 1, 2020.

5 Proclamation on Suspension of Entry as Immigrants and Nonimmigrants of Persons who Pose a Risk of

Transmitting 2019 Novel Coronavirus HEALTH-CARE Issued on: January 31, 2020. https://www.whitehouse.gov/presidential-actions/proclamation-suspension-entry-immigrants-nonimmigrants-persons-pose-risk-transmitting-2019-novel-coronavirus/. Accessed Nov. 1, 2020.

6 Strang, Stephen. God, Trump, and COVID-19: How the Pandemic Is Affecting Christians, the World, and America's 2020 Election (p. xi). Charisma House. Kindle Edition.

7 Domenico Cucinotta, Maurizio Vanelli. WHO Declares COVID-19 a Pandemic 2020 Mar 19;91(1):157-160. doi: 10.23750/abm. v91i1.9397. https://pubmed.ncbi.nlm.nih.gov/32191675/#:~:text=The%20World%20Health%20Organization%20(,outbreak%20a%20global%20pandemic. Accessed Nov. 15, 2020.

8 Naomi Florea Buda. October 31, 2020, posted on social media FB. TRIAL SITE NEWS.COM. This man has COVID. He has a plan. For all of us.

9 Pathophysiological Basis and Rationale for Early Outpatient Treatment of SARS-CoV-2 (COVID-19) Infection. The American Journal of Medicine, 7 August 2020. https://www.sciencedirect.com/science/article/pii/S0002934320306732. Accessed Nov. 15, 2020.

10 https://aapsonline.org/covid-19-fdas-negativism-on-hcq-is-unfounded/. Accessed Nov. 2020.

11 Ronan J. Kelly, MD, et. al. Pathophysiological Basis and Rationale for Early Outpatient Treatment of SARS-CoV-2 (COVID-19) Infection. The American Journal of Medicine, 7 August 2020. https://www.sciencedirect.com/science/article/pii/S0002934320306732. Accessed Nov. 15, 2020.

12 https://www.bbc.com/news/world-us-cana-

da-53575964. Accessed Nov. 20, 2020.

13 https://www.bbc.com/news/51980731. Accessed Nov. 20, 2020.

14 Ibid.

15 Andrew Mark Miller. Study finds 84% fewer hospitalizations for patients treated with controversial drug hydroxychloroquine. Washington Examiner | November 25, 2020 03:02 PM. https://www.washingtonexaminer.com/news/study-finds-84-fewer-hospitalizations-for-patients-treated-with-controversial-drug-hydroxychloroquine. Accessed Dec. 10, 2020.

16 https://www.bakersfield.com/news/local-doctors-featured-in-viral-video-of-doctors-that-was-later-banned-from-social-media/article_fd9da404-d8ec-11ea-aeae-47e7e993c84d.html. Accessed Dec. 10, 2020.

17 Brian Tyson, MD. The Miracle of the Imperial Valley: Dr. Tyson's first-person account of COVID-19. The Desert Review. Nov. 1, 2020. https://www.thedesertreview.com/news/the-miracle-of-the-imperial-valley-dr-tyson-s-first-person-account-of-covid-19/article_a8707136-196b-11eb-bc7b-87d7730460bb.html. Accessed Dec. 10, 2020.

18 Strang, Stephen. God, Trump, and COVID-19: How the Pandemic Is Affecting Christians, the World, and America's 2020 Election (p. 64). Charisma House. Kindle Edition.

19 Vinay Prasad, MD, MPH. Op-Ed: What Does 'Follow the Science' Mean, Anyway?—Science is a tool, not a prescription for policy on COVID-19. MedPage Today, November 23, 2020. medpagetoday.com/blogs/vinay-pr…

20 https://docs.google.com/document/d/1E9ZxEOJ6nH6C4qE8KEF8byt1LYqkGorOoI2ZQwAKml0/edit.

Coronavirus Article Archive. Articles on COVID-19 to Share with Patients, Colleagues, the Media, and others (sorted by date published). Accessed Dec. 15, 2020.

21 https://aapsonline.org/covid-19-fdas-negativism-on-hcq-is-unfounded/. Accessed Dec. 15, 2020.

22 Ibid.

23 Harvey Risch. FDA obstruction: Patients die, while Trump gets the blame. October 19, 2020. https://www.washingtonexaminer.com/opinion/fda-obstruction-patients-die-while-trump-gets-the-blame?_amp=true&__twitter_impression=true. Accessed Dec. 15, 2020.

24 https://www.preprints.org/manuscript/202007.0025/v1. https://www.sciencedirect.com/science/article/pii/S0924857920304258. Accessed Dec. 20, 2020.

25 COVID-19 outpatients – early risk-stratified treatment with zinc plus low-dose hydroxychloroquine and azithromycin: a retrospective case series study. International Journal of Antimicrobial Agents. Available online 26 October 2020. https://www.sciencedirect.com/science/article/pii/S0924857920304258. Accessed Dec. 20, 2020.

26 Dr. Vladimir Zelenko. Zelenko Protocol: Treatment Plan for Patients with COVID-19 symptoms. Prehospital Management. Twitter: @zev_dr. https://docs.google.com/document/d/1TaRDwXMhQHSMsgrs9TFBclHjPHerXMuB87DUXmcAvwg/edit. Accessed Nov. 14, 2020.

27 Mary Beth Pfeiffer. This Doctor has COVID-19. He has a plan. For all of us. OCT 30, 2020 | BLOG, NEWS, POPULAR POSTS, TSN NEWS. TrailSiteNews.com. Accessed Nov. 15, 2020.

28 Review of the Emerging Evidence Supporting the

Efficacy of Ivermectin in the Prophylaxis and Treatment of COVID-19 [FLCCC Alliance; updated Jan 12, 2021] 2 / 30. www.flccc.net. Accessed Jan. 20, 2021.

29 Review of the Emerging Evidence Demonstrating the Efficacy of Ivermectin in the Prophylaxis and Treatment of COVID-19. Pierre Kory, MD, G. Umberto Meduri, MD, Jose Iglesias, DO, Joseph Varon, MD, Keith Berkowitz, MD, Howard Kornfeld, MD, Eivind Vinjevoll, MD, Scott Mitchell, MBChB, Fred Wagshul, MD, Paul E. Marik, MD. https://covid-19criticalcare.com/i-mask-prophylaxis-treatment-protocol/faq-on-ivermectin. Accessed February 09, 2021.

30 Angela Betsaida B. Laguipo, BSN. Oct 9 2020. "86 percent of the UK's COVID-19 patients have no symptoms." News Medical Life Science. https://www.news-medical.net/news/20201009/86-percent-of-the-UKs-COVID-19-patients-have-no-symptoms.aspx. Accessed November 14, 2020.

31 https://www.cdc.gov/coronavirus/2019-ncov/symptoms-testing/symptoms.html#seek-medical-attention. Accessed Jan. 15, 2020.

32 Cathy C. Blaylock. Face Masks Pose Serious Risks to the Healthy. June 11, 2020. Coronavirus COVID-19 Education. https://theplantstrongclub.org/2020/06/11/dr-russell-blaylock-face-masks-pose-serious-risks-to-the-healthy/. Accessed Nov. 20, 2020.

33 https://www.cdc.gov/coronavirus/2019-ncov/symptoms-testing/symptoms.html#seek-medical-attention. Accessed Oct. 10, 2020.

34 Ibid.

35 Crandall, Dr. Chauncey. Fight Back (p.72, 73). Hu-

manix Books. Kindle Edition.

36 Ibid.

37 Crandall, Dr. Chauncey. Fight Back (p. 8). Humanix Books. Kindle Edition.

38 Cathy C. Blaylock. Face Masks Pose Serious Risks to the Healthy. June 11, 2020. Coronavirus CO-VID-19, Education. https://theplantstrongclub. org/2020/06/11/dr-russell-blaylock-face-masks-pose-serious-risks-to-the-healthy/. Accessed Nov. 30, 2020.

39 Dr. Rodica Malos. Find Your Peace: Supernatural Solutions Beyond Science for Fear, Anxiety, and Depression. Lake Mary Florida: Siloam. Charisma Media/Charisma House Book Group. February, 2020.

40 Dr. Scott Hannen. Stop the Pain: The Six to Fix. 2019. Trilogy Publishing Group. Tustin, CA.

41 Judy George. 80% of COVID-19 Patients May Have Lingering Symptoms, Signs— More Than 50 Effects Persisted After Acute Infection, Meta-analysis Shows by Judy George, Senior Staff Writer, MedPage Today. January 30, 2021.

42 Rita Rubin. As Their Numbers Grow, CO-VID-19 "Long Haulers" Stump Experts. Medical News & Perspectives. September 23, 2020. JAMA. 2020;324(14):1381-1383. doi:10.1001/jama.2020.17709

43 https://www.cdc.gov/coronavirus/2019-ncov/long-term-effects.html. Accessed February 10, 2021.

44 Fact Sheet for Recipients and Caregivers: Emergency Use Authorization (EUA) of the Pfizer-BioNTech COVID-19 Vaccine to Prevent Coronavirus Disease 2019 (COVID-19) in Individuals 16 Years of Age and Older. Pfizer-BioNTech COVID-19 Vaccine EUA Fact Sheet for ... – FDA. www.fda.gov. Accessed Feb.

10, 2020.

45 https://www.hackensackmeridianhealth.org/
HealthU/2021/01/11/a-simple-breakdown-of-the-
ingredients-in-the-covid-vaccines/. Accessed Feb. 10,
2020.

46 Serena Marshall and Lara Salahi. What Do We
Really Know About Pfizer's New COVID-19
Vax?— Answers from Pfizer exec Phil Dormitzer. MedPage Today. December 16, 2020.
https://www.medpagetoday.com/podcasts/
trackthevax/90243?xid=nl_mpt_DHE_2020-12
17&eun=g1679824d0r&utm_source=Sailthru&utm_
medium=email&utm_campaign=Daily%20Head-
lines%20Top%20Cat%20HeC%20%202020-12
17&utm_term=NL_Daily_DHE_dual-gmail-defini-
tion. Accessed Feb. 9, 2021.

47 Dr. Simona Dehelean, Pharm. D. Texas.

48 Understanding and Explaining mRNA COVID-19
Vaccines | CDC Accessed March 24, 2021.

49 Rumiana Tenchov. Understanding the nanotechnology in COVID-19 vaccines. Posted February 18,
2021. Understanding the nanotechnology in CO-
VID-19 vaccines | CAS. Accessed March 24, 2021.

50 Dr. Scott Hannen. Stop the Pain: The Six to Fix. 2019
(p. 270). Trilogy Publishing Group. Tustin, CA.

51 https://christiancivics.org/podcast/prayer-from-the-
front-lines-of-corona-virus-research/.

52 Dr. Scott Hannen. Stop the Pain: The Six to Fix. 2019
(p. 270-271). Trilogy Publishing Group. Tustin, CA.

53 https://www.nytimes.com/2020/03/31/us/politics/
coronavirus-death-toll-united-states.html.

54 C.H. Spurgeon. Prayer (p. 125).

55 Strang, Stephen . God, Trump, and COVID-19: How
the Pandemic Is Affecting Christians, the World, and

America's 2020 Election (p. 62). Charisma House. Kindle Edition.

56 Dr. Rodica Malos. Created in His Image with Unique Purpose: Science and Beyond, Holy Spirit is Real. Trilogy/TBN, 2021.

57 Dr. Rodica Malos, Find Your Peace: Supernatural Solutions Beyond Science for Fear, Anxiety, and Depression (p. 267). Lake Mary Florida: Siloam. Charisma Media/Charisma House Book Group, 2020.

58 Ronan J. Kelly, MD, et al. Pathophysiological Basis and Rationale for Early Outpatient Treatment of SARS-CoV-2 (COVID-19) Infection. The American Journal of Medicine, 7 August 2020. https://www.sciencedirect.com/science/article/pii/S0002934320306732. Accessed Nov. 15, 2020.

CPSIA information can be obtained
at www.ICGtesting.com
Printed in the USA
LVHW050909030621
689238LV00015B/642